Praise for
Before the Change

"The single best book you can read on cooperating with nature as your body shifts gears in preparation for the powerful menopausal years."

—Joan Borysenko, Ph.D., author of *Minding the Body, Mending the Mind* and *A Woman's Book of Life*

"American natural health doyenne Ann Louise Gittleman describes the changes women experience before the change and presents a program for countering unpleasant symptoms."

—*Natural Health*

"Loaded with exactly the kind of information women need to support their bodies during perimenopause."

—Christiane Northrup, M.D., author of *Women's Bodies, Women's Wisdom*

Before the
the
Change

Also by Ann Louise Gittleman, Ph.D., C.N.S.

BOOKS

The New Fat Flush Plan
Fat Flush for Life
The Complete Fat Flush Program
The New Fat Flush Cookbook
The New Fat Flush Foods
The New Fat Flush Journal and Shopping Guide
The New Fat Flush Fitness Plan
Zapped
The Gut Flush Plan
The Fast Track Detox Diet
Hot Times
Ann Louise Gittleman's Guide to the 40/30/30 Phenomenon
Eat Fat, Lose Weight Cookbook
The Living Beauty Detox Program
Why Am I Always So Tired?
Super Nutrition for Men
How to Stay Young and Healthy in a Toxic World
Eat Fat, Lose Weight
Overcoming Parasites
Super Nutrition for Menopause
Beyond Probiotics
The 40/30/30 Phenomenon
Your Body Knows Best
Get the Salt Out
Get the Sugar Out
Guess What Came to Dinner? Parasites and Your Health
Super Nutrition for Women
Beyond Pritikin

ELECTRONIC MEDIA

Eat Fat, Lose Weight for Kindle
The Fat Flush App for iPhone and iPad

Before
the
Change

Taking Charge of Your
PERIMENOPAUSE

Ann Louise Gittleman, Ph.D., C.N.S.

HarperOne
An Imprint of HarperCollins*Publishers*

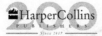

This book contains advice and information relating to health care. It should be used to supplement rather than replace the advice of your doctor or another trained health professional. If you know or suspect you have a health problem, it is recommended that you seek your physician's advice before embarking on any medical program or treatment. All efforts have been made to ensure the accuracy of the information contained in this book as of the date of publication. This publisher and the author disclaim liability for any medical outcomes that may occur as a result of applying the methods suggested in this book.

All names, without exception, have been changed to protect the identities of the women involved.

HarperCollins books may be purchased for educational, business, or sales promotional use. For information, please email the Special Markets Department at SPsales@harpercollins.com.

FIRST HARPERCOLLINS PAPERBACK EDITION PUBLISHED IN 1998. Revised and updated in 2003 and 2017.

Designed by SBI Book Arts, LLC

Library of Congress Cataloging-in-Publication Data has been applied for.

ISBN 978–0–06–264231–8

17 18 19 20 21   LSC   10 9 8 7 6 5 4 3 2 1

To all the courageous women everywhere who
are entering a brand-new stage of life

Contents

Acknowledgments

Many times a day I realize how much my own
life is built on the labors of my fellow men, and
how earnestly I must exert myself in order to
give in return as much as I have received.

—ALBERT EINSTEIN

I especially want to acknowledge the remarkable women who have influenced my life and touched my heart in very profound ways. These women have all passed and are no doubt entertaining the angels. The list of these "women of valor" includes my mother, Edith; my teacher, alternative medicine's grande dame Dr. Hazel Parcells; my herbal healing guru, Hanna Kroeger; my personal friends the great Gracie Aldworth, Ann Oliphant, Wilma Keller, and Dr. Ann Wigmore; the unforgettable Barbara Carmichael; Jane Murray Heimlich (the daughter of the dancing great and wife of the doctor who invented the "Heimlich maneuver"); and Sondra Metzger. Not a day goes by that I don't think about one of you.

And my heartfelt gratitude to the other women who have personally changed my life with their open hearts and outrageous graciousness: the one and only Gloria Bein, Susan Meredith, and the legendary Patricia Bragg.

The late screen star Gloria Swanson was also a personal friend of mine and a true health pioneer, years ahead of her time.

I'd also like to extend my heartfelt gratitude to the whole hardworking team at HarperCollins, including Hilary Lawson, Sydney Rogers, Adia Colar, Julia Kent, and Adrian Morgan.

Grateful thanks to the entire HarperOne team, especially Gideon Weil, Mary Duke, and the entire publicity team. Finally, kudos to my ALG team on the home front, including Ally Mortensen, Stuart Gittleman, Emily Carmichael, Carol Templeton Volanski, and Shae Janda. A special shout-out to my tireless and terrific literary agent, Coleen O'Shea, who has been with me throughout my career. Love you all!

Preface

"I'm just too young for this!"

These may be the most frequently spoken words you will hear yourself say as you begin your menopausal journey during your thirties and forties (and for some, the journey may begin as early as your late twenties). This time in your life is when a whole host of environmental, dietary, and lifestyle factors seem to conspire against your body, creating an array of seemingly disconnected and utterly annoying symptoms. Among them: mood swings, a lagging sex drive, sleeplessness, exhaustion, GI woes, belly fat, hot flashes, depression, and a sluggish metabolism.

It has been almost twenty years since I wrote the first edition of this book. Since then, the perimenopausal landscape has greatly evolved.

In 2002, the Women's Health Initiative, a major national long-term study involving hormone replacement therapy, which was the go-to treatment for women during the menopausal years, was abruptly halted. The study had utilized a combination of popular synthetic hormones called Prempro (a mix of estrogen and progestin). Why was the study halted? In the initial stages of the research it became clear that the risks of hormone use far outweighed the benefits. Those risks included a 26 percent greater chance of breast cancer, a 41 percent higher rate of stroke, a 29 percent greater risk of heart disease, and double the rate of blood clots in the legs and lungs. Women were frantic and scared, with many questions and concerns about the synthetic hormone replacement therapy (HRT) they had been on for years or were contemplating. Many felt they no longer had any safe treatment options for the symptoms of perimenopause—what ideally should be a natural and freeing transition into a brand-new phase of life. So only five years after the initial printing of *Before the Change,* I felt compelled to update the first edition with a section on the pros and cons of hormone therapy as well as how to wean off the synthetics and transition to more natural, bioidentical hormone treatments. After all, hormones are the chemical messengers of the body. They influence everything we think, feel, and do. In spite of that, we don't know much more about their intricate workings than we do about the surface of Mars. The more we learn about hormones, the more we find how little we know.

In the first update, I expanded upon the pros and cons of phyto-hormones (like soy) and offered new insights into bioidentical hormones as effective and safe alternatives to HRT. Bioidentical hormones are the real deal: hormones that are identical to what the female body has been producing naturally for roughly two hundred thousand years. They are far different biochemically from the hormones found in Premarin, the common HRT made from hormones concentrated in horse urine. They are also far different from Provera, or medroxyprogesterone, the synthetic progesterone that is harmful to a woman's heart.

After an appearance on *Dr. Phil*, which swept *Before the Change* onto the *New York Times* bestseller list, I continued to hear from women everywhere who had more questions that the first updated edition hadn't addressed. They needed advice about frustrating weight gain, leaky gut syndrome, fibromyalgia, chronic fatigue, polycystic ovary syndrome (PCOS), Hashimoto's thyroiditis, and what to do to restore balance after a hysterectomy. They were concerned about breast health, bone strength, signs of accelerated aging, and a relatively new area of study: pelvic floor dysfunction. I felt all these women deserved drug-free, proactive solutions to their problems, or, at the very least, some type of direction as to where to go for proper care.

Many of these issues are now discussed in chapter 14, "Secret Cures for Perimenopause Problems." Throughout the book I also answer the most prevalent questions I was asked over and over again during the past two decades:

While bioidentical hormones may be natural, are they always safe?

You'll be surprised to learn that large quantities of bioidentical estrogens, for example, can increase the risk of blood clots and stroke. I'll tell you how to avoid estrogen-related blood clots easily and entirely.

What are the latest findings about calcium? Is supplementation of calcium still the gold standard to prevent osteoporosis?

I'll discuss the reasons that calcium is no longer the go-to remedy for thinning bones and why magnesium, "vitamin" D (which is actually a hormone), vitamin K2, and strontium are your bones' besties. Research now suggests that calcium can cause arterial congestion, digestive issues, calcification in cancerous tumors, and many more unwanted conditions.

Why can't I lose weight?

You'll be astonished to find out that hypothyroidism is now approaching epidemic proportions among perimenopausal women, and most women go undiagnosed. In this new edition of *Before the Change,* you'll find updated and expanded discussions of the gluten–thyroid connection, the role of bile, how thyroid function relates to hormonal imbalances, why your doctor can't tell you what's wrong, and what you can do to keep your thyroid in tip-top shape.

In addition, you'll discover a brand-new "Peri Zapper"—my tried-and-true remedies for perimenopausal symptoms—that focuses on a properly nourished liver (the liver's production of quality bile is absolutely essential for optimum hormone support) as well as a whole-body detoxification. This, in and of itself, may be the *most* important way to help your body navigate the "change before the change."

I'm so glad you have picked up this book. (I wish I'd had this type of guide when I was experiencing perimenopause.) You have joined the millions of women going through these changes. By learning how to balance your lifestyle habits, tweak your diet to utilize nutrients, and implement the Peri exercises and herbal and bioidentical hormone remedies, you'll discover the very best options for your health—before, during, and even after menopause. Get ready for the most exciting new phase of your life!

Before the Change

1.

You're Not Crazy! It's Just Perimenopause!

Discovering the Root Cause Behind Symptoms You Didn't Even Know Were Related

I remember it well.

At the age of forty-seven, after a productive but extremely stressful year of travel, radio shows, lectures, and book promotions, I had relocated my office and was in the midst of remodeling my home. While the pressure of all these activities had propelled me to a new level of stress and tension, I kept reminding myself that in the past I had thrived under pressure. Back then, no matter how much stress I had been under—from manuscript deadlines to public appearances in front of thousands of people—once my head hit that pillow, I was out and always slept through the night. But this age was different.

Something was definitely changing in my body. I began to imagine the possibility of never getting a good night's sleep again, and that made me feel even more anxious and depressed.

It wasn't until I took an entire battery of blood tests, including an FSH (follicle-stimulating hormone) indicator, that it dawned on me what was really happening. I was smack-dab in perimenopause. But my concept of what this meant was purely academic. I knew that it was a time of about ten years in a woman's life during which her body changes its secretion and processing of the hormones needed for reproduction. Two months earlier, for the first time in my life, I had missed a period, but I'd attributed it to excessive travel and the body clock adjustments that come with flying through various time zones.

Yet it was also true that over the past ten years I had become noticeably more irritable and less patient—with a shorter fuse—and I had developed a shorter attention span. I had attributed these personality changes to my increased focus on work. It had never once occurred to me that something biochemical, such as hormones, was changing in my body, affecting my nervous system. To further confound the situation, I didn't have any telltale symptoms, like hot flashes or night sweats.

Nevertheless, I finally connected the dots between my disconcerting symptoms and their cause. If only I had recognized earlier what my body was trying to tell me, I would have sought remedies much sooner. Those ten years could have been far more pleasurable for me than they were. I say this even though my symptoms were not as severe as those suffered by many women during their perimenopause.

Motivated by my own experience, I set out on a mission to enlighten women everywhere between the ages of thirty-five and fifty about this newly recognized stage of life called perimenopause. In addition to comparing notes with women from this age group, I attended perimenopause conferences, reviewed special publications, and interviewed doctors, psychologists, researchers, and product developers. I also personally experimented with a variety of remedies based on state-of-the-art comprehensive hormone profiles.

What I learned was appalling. The scant information available on perimenopause was frequently incomplete and misleading, and the treatments highly risky to follow. U.S. women are still being told to take antianxiety medication and sleeping pills for disturbed sleeping patterns—symptoms caused by the new norm of perimenopausal hormonal imbalances. In fact, antidepressants are the third most frequently taken medication in the United States, because they are now prescribed for a variety of maladies, including natural perimenopause-related anxiety and depression, and hormonal disruptions like premenstrual syndrome (PMS). Researchers are taking it a step further and investigating the use of antidepressants to treat other premenopausal symptoms, like hot flashes.

Meanwhile, millions of women never discover the fundamental cause of their emotional and physical symptoms. As Dr. Nancy Lee Teaff, author of *Perimenopause: Preparing for the Change,* told *New Woman* magazine, "Skipped periods and hot flashes are almost automatically attributed to menopause, but if your first symptom happens to be insomnia, you may spend hours in a therapist's office before it becomes apparent that the problem is primarily hormonal."

Perimenopause Symptoms

Acne	Insomnia
Allergies	Irritability
Anger	Joint pain
Ankles or feet swelling	Leg cramps
Anxiety	Memory problems
Backache	Menstrual cycle irregularities
Bloating	Migraines
Blood sugar imbalance	Mood swings
Blood sugar level reduction	Muscular weakness
Bone loss	Night sweats
Breast sagging	Panic attacks
Breast tenderness	Sexual desire loss
Depression	Skin aging and dryness
Facial hair	Skin itching and crawling
Fatigue	Skin spots (liver or age spots)
Feelings of being crazy	Stomach cramps
Fibrocystic breasts	Urinary incontinence
Fuzzy thinking	Urinary infections
Hair loss or thinning	Uterine fibroids
Headaches	Vaginal dryness
Heart palpitations	Water retention
Hot flashes	Weeping
Hypothyroidism	Weight gain
Hysteria	Weight loss inability

During perimenopause, as with menopause, the ovaries become less active and the body prepares to stop menstruating. One of the primary hormones affected by this is estrogen. Many neurotransmitters depend upon estrogen to maintain normal functioning. As a result, changes in estrogen levels have far-reaching effects beyond the purely physical manifestations, including problems with sleep, memory, and cognitive function. These help to create the feeling of "being in a fog" that so many women experience during perimenopause.

Additionally, emotional and physical symptoms fluctuate greatly when hormones and brain chemistry vacillate. Think of the uniquely female experience after childbirth, and during perimenopause and menopause. Stressful, right? When the stressors of daily life are added to the mix, neurotransmitter imbalances are amplified, and we can become more high-strung.

As we desperately seek new remedies for these perimenopausal symptoms, we often look in all the wrong places. We—like I did in my forties—mistakenly try to treat each symptom as a separate problem; instead, we need to discover the single underlying thread. Once we restore greater balance to our hormones, our symptoms usually fade and may even disappear on their own, as happened in my life. But to accomplish this, we have to recognize the connection between symptoms and hormones—and make that association before midlife hormone changes take their mental, physical, and emotional toll. Many of us are presently in this situation. And that's why I had to write this book.

PMS or Perimenopause?

Perimenopause often feels like a bad case of premenstrual syndrome (PMS). Indeed, many of the symptoms are the same due to similar hormonal shifts that occur. During both perimenopause and PMS, estrogen and progesterone levels change, causing bloating, weight gain, food cravings, headaches, depression, irritability, lack of energy, and loss of concentration—but more on this later.

How can you tell the difference? Apply this simple rule: If your periods continue to occur regularly, it's PMS. If your periods are irregular, it's perimenopause.

Although you can miss your period for a variety of reasons, including pregnancy, a continuing but irregular monthly cycle is a strong reason to suspect that you have a hormonal imbalance, which, depending on your age, can very well be due to perimenopause.

Think of perimenopause as a second puberty (despite any negative high school memories that may evoke). Like puberty, and many other normal biological shifts, perimenopause is gradual—or, as some might say, insidious—and it causes unpleasant symptoms if your body is out of whack. Many women notice a pattern of "worsening PMS," starting as early as in their late twenties, which is probably the beginning of early ovarian hormonal shifts leading to perimenopause.

Quiz:
Are You in Perimenopause?

Perimenopause should not be thought of as a disease or treated like one. It's a naturally occurring transition before the change. You can alleviate its symptoms in various ways, depending on how far along in the transition you are presently. Your answers to these questions will help you decide on your current status.

Scoring

Place the appropriate number in the Score column according to the intensity or frequency of your symptoms.

- Symptom is mild or occasional: 1

- Symptom is moderate or frequent: 2

- Symptom is severe: 3

Questions

After answering all ten questions, add up your total score.

SCORE

1. Do you feel depressed or have the "blues"   _____
   for no apparent reason?

2. Do you experience restlessness, irritability,   _____
   and/or anxiety?

3. Have your sleep patterns changed, with frequent awakenings or insomnia? _____

4. Does your heart sometimes pound while you are resting or sitting? _____

5. Do you have food cravings? _____

6. Do you have bloating or fluid retention? _____

7. Do you need to urinate more frequently? _____

8. Has your sex drive diminished? _____

9. Do you often have headaches or migraines? _____

10. Are you starting to put on weight around the middle? _____

TOTAL SCORE _____

If your total score is between 10 and 18: Don't worry, you're not going crazy. You're probably just beginning the perimenopause transition. A hormone-regulating diet, supplements, regular moderate exercise, and better management of stress may be all you need to alleviate your symptoms.

If your total score is between 19 and 28: Diet, exercise, and stress management may or may not be enough to alleviate your symptoms. Additional nutrients and natural progesterone cream should make all the difference.

If your total score is above 28: You're fully in perimenopause. The remedies mentioned for the lower scores may be sufficient. If they're not, consider taking natural hormones. But first have a saliva test to determine your hormone levels.

At What Age Will You Reach Menopause?

The Greek words *men pausis* mean "month to end," and *peri* means "near." Both perimenopause and menopause are stages in a longer process known as the climacteric, which encompasses the hormonal changes in a woman's body that take place from about age thirty-five to about age sixty. The average age of menopause for U.S. women is fifty-one, but perimenopausal symptoms are felt by some women who are only thirty-five years old.

Is there any way to tell at what age you will reach menopause? Your most likely age is your mother's age when she reached menopause. Heredity is important in this, but other factors are influential too. Therefore, the more your health and lifestyle resemble those of your mother, the likelier it will be that heredity will be the deciding factor. The accompanying chart shares some factors that can contribute to an earlier onset of menopause. If many of these factors apply to your mother in her forties but not to you, you may reach menopause at a later age than she did. Unfortunately, the reverse also holds true. If more of these factors apply to you now than did to her in her forties, you may reach menopause earlier than she did.

Early Menopause Factors

	Your Mother	You
Anorexic or bulimic		
Cholesterol level below normal		
Cigarette smoker		
Lower socioeconomic background		
Never had children		
Ovaries medically irritated		
Overweight		
Pituitary gland problems		
Strict vegetarian		
Very thin athlete (especially marathon runner)		

In the United States, generally speaking, women who bear a child after the age of forty and white women of northern European, African, or Mediterranean or southern European origin reach menopause at a later age than other women. In some women, menopause can be abrupt. In others, at the opposite extreme, it can be a gradual transition occurring between about age thirty-five and age fifty. Both ends of the spectrum are perfectly normal and healthy.

Individual perimenopausal differences among women do not reflect their comparative states of health. A woman can be extremely healthy and genetically or otherwise predisposed to perimenopausal symptoms. We need to keep in mind that perimenopause is part of a natural process, not a pathological one.

In the United States alone, approximately seventy million women are experiencing some aspect of "the change." Despite this huge number, the medical community has only begun to recognize perimenopause over the past decade as a distinct stage of a woman's life. Most members of this community—including ob-gyns and endocrinologists—spend just one to two hours of their medical training learning about menopause and sexual education. Since so many physicians are still not aware of perimenopause, of course they do not recognize moodiness, anxiety, weight gain, fuzzy thinking, or depression as its symptoms.

Which Hormones?

Once you have made the connection between your symptoms and hormones, it's easy to fall into a common trap. Instead of wondering exactly which hormones are causing your symptoms, you may assume that female sex hormones alone lie behind all your problems. However, stress hormones as well as environmental hormone-disrupting chemical culprits are likely in cahoots with the sex hormones. In fact, for those of you in your late twenties, thirties, or forties with symptoms for which a hormone imbalance is a likely cause, you need to consider five different hormone systems. Of course, these five hormone systems are all interconnected in the body, and they influence one another in countless ways, but it may be easier to think of them separately as follows:

Blood Sugar Hormones		
Glucagon	Insulin	

Stress Hormones		
Adrenaline	Cortisol	

Sex Hormones		
Estrogen	Progesterone	Testosterone

Hunger Hormones		
Adiponectin	Ghrelin	Leptin

Antiaging Hormone		
Human growth hormone		

Among the five groups, there is an obvious relationship between nutrition, stress, lifestyle, and sex hormones. (Both the adrenal glands and the ovaries secrete sex hormones.) One thing has constantly reminded me of this relationship: the high number of complaints from women who have had hormone replacement therapy. These women continually report that they don't feel right, even after their symptoms have subsided. I consider this alongside the reality that the vast majority of women stop taking prescription hormones within five years because they feel better without them.

The only way I know for your body to feel right is to keep all therapeutic procedures as noninvasive and natural as possible. A balanced diet is the most healthful, cost-effective, and enjoyable form of therapy. Most enlightened or integrative functional medicine physicians would not be surprised to learn that what initially looked like a perimenopause symptom disappeared when the patient was placed on a balanced diet.

What I have observed many, many times is that women with imbalances of blood sugar or stress hormones have symptoms that are often indistinguishable from perimenopause symptoms. When these women eat a better diet or learn to manage their stress more effectively, they often are "miraculously" cured of their perimenopause symptoms at the same time. Coincidence? I think not.

First, Do No Harm

The Hippocratic Oath, taken by all medical school students upon graduation, reads, "First, do no harm."

As a professional nutritionist and functional medicine advocate, I have dedicated much of my career to teaching and prescribing nutritional therapy for female health problems. Not so many years ago, shockingly few people—including women themselves—were willing to give priority to either female health problems or nutrition. Today, more and more individuals look for an underlying cause and find that the cause may very well *be the cure*.

Although this book is mainly about how women can use nutritional therapy for perimenopausal symptoms, I do *not* feel that nutrition or bioidentical hormone replacement therapy alone are always right for everybody. In fact, for some women there may be a period of time, known as the "estrogen window," in which estrogen replacement may be advised. This may be especially true for women who have had a hysterectomy and are no longer producing any estrogen, resulting in a need to shore up levels quickly and at higher amounts.

That being said, when food, nutritional supplements, stress relief, and other lifestyle changes can be successfully implemented, most women can ameliorate their hormone-related discomfort without any hormone replacement therapy at all. If your body can heal itself in a natural way, my interpretation of the Hippocratic Oath would argue against introducing something artificial into your body.

This especially holds true for synthetic hormone replacement therapy. It has been linked to cancer through multiple studies, most significantly the landmark Women's Health Initiative—as mentioned in the new preface. From my nutritionist perspective, "do no harm" means using the least invasive, most naturally healing solution to any health concern or uncomfortable symptoms. Perimenopause is no exception.

Changing How We Think About the Change

The diet world has been turned upside down with the awareness that the foods we eat cause a hormonal response inside the body. In this book, I use this knowledge to turn your world right side up by applying it to the hormonal imbalances that occur during perimenopause. I review the hormonal responses that macronutrients (carbohydrates, protein, and fat) and environmental agents (xenoestrogens) evoke in your body, and utilize them to restore hormonal functioning during this changing time.

I have a big fat surprise for you: eating fat does not make you fat. As I have been advising my readers and my clients for more than thirty-five years, nothing could be further from the truth. The right fats, which I call your "sexy, slimming fats," actually reset hormones, reduce inflammation, and fix metabolism. In addition, fats assist in reprogramming the stress, sex, and hunger hormones that can exacerbate perimenopause symptoms and cause weight gain. So not only does fat not make you fat, but fat also makes you skinny!

However, it's not enough to just eat fat, lose weight, and manufacture hormones. Your body needs to be able to process that fat—which is where your liver and bile come in. I will teach you how to support your liver and optimize its bile production. Bile is the fluid the liver produces daily to break down fats into a digestible form and transport excess water out of the body. Poor-quality bile is a newly discovered factor in hypothyroidism. Better bile means fewer digestive woes, like constipation, bloating, and gas, and fewer hypothyroid-like symptoms, like fatigue, weight gain, and brain fog. This may be a godsend for anyone who does not have a gallbladder and therefore lacks the storage tank that regulates the properly timed secretion of bile when eating fat. For these individuals, bile replacement is a necessity.

In this book we also examine several key nutrients that every woman must have in the correct amounts in order to feel emotionally and physically well. My professional experience has shown that women are most likely to be deficient in certain nutrients, such as magnesium, zinc, and the B vitamins, and that every woman must have these in the correct dosage in order to feel emotionally and physically well. Magnesium, for example, has even been called the "original chill pill," acting as a hormone balancer and relieving anxiety, constipation, or any ailment where an overstimulation of the nervous system is present.

I would be remiss if I didn't include moderate exercise too, which helps all hormone systems to function better and reduces stress. Indeed, exercise contributes positively to just about every bodily function and to most emotional and intellectual functions as well. Exercising for at least four hours a week lowers estrogen dominance (when skipped periods result in low progesterone levels), reduces cortisol levels, and supports bone health, all of which will make the perimenopause period pass more smoothly. I am especially a fan of high-intensity interval training (HIIT), rebounding, and the Power Plate (see Resources for more information), all of which you will read more about later in this book. The secret of a good exercise program is to find something that you enjoy doing and that fits conveniently into your daily schedule. The more preparation that exercise requires, the easier it will be to find a reason to skip it. But if you do something simple that you enjoy, you will want to do it every day. I will share with you how to exercise effectively, efficiently, and enjoyably.

I cannot emphasize enough the role stress plays in perimenopause. Simply dealing with your unique manifestation of perimenopause symptoms constitutes a stressful experience. Add the stresses encountered in daily life, and your body may very well find itself struggling to keep up. When you are chronically stressed, it exacerbates perimenopause symptoms and leaves you with a whole array of other issues. The adrenals can become exhausted and cortisol levels can become erratic. This causes most bodily functions to slow down, thus your body is not operating at its full potential. This also means your body is not as well equipped to handle hormonal fluctuations, further intensifying your symptoms of both stress and perimenopause. I will show you how to tame the cortisol monster through healing oils, exercise, sleep, and coping skills.

Eating a hormone-regulating diet, exercising moderately on a regular basis, and managing daily stress is often enough to alleviate the discomfort and symptoms felt by many women in their thirties and forties. However, diet, exercise, and stress management may not always be enough. You may need to resort to natural hormone therapy.

Natural progesterone is usually the key therapeutic hormone, rather than estrogen. Natural progesterone creams are available over the counter without a prescription, and I will list my favorite brands for you. I also look at phytohormones (hormones from plants) and explain why they work.

In cases where not even natural progesterone cream and phyto-hormones are enough to alleviate the symptoms, you may need to implement bioidentical hormones, compounded specially on an in-dividual basis. However, whether these are bioidentical hormones or their synthetic substitutes, all hormones need to be monitored by a practitioner, especially bioidentical estrogen. Ultimately, all hormones are broken down by the liver. That's why liver support is key, and one of the central features of my Peri program.

The balance of this book is devoted to the principles of the Peri Prescription, a hormone-regulating eating plan that women need for their twenties, thirties, forties, and beyond. After I share with you the science behind what makes this powerful diet so necessary, I will give you a meal plan and recipes to help you get started. Keep in mind that this is not a one-diet-fits-all food plan. It can be tailored for individ-ual differences based upon ancestry, metabolic rate, blood type, and dietary restrictions. The diet is varied and fun—with a manageable shopping list!

To start you off, though, and to help steady you along your hor-monal journey, the following chapter introduces ten highly effective Peri Zappers to rescue you from perimenopausal symptoms and give you your life back. These ten remedies are recommended because they are especially reliable, usually free of side effects, and easy to use. Peri Zappers help balance the levels of all types of hormones, and I will dis-cuss how to use them to alleviate symptoms, feel fit and trim, and lead a more harmonious life.

Perimenopause can be a major challenge. But, as with any challenge women have faced over the course of their lives and the course of his-tory, you will experience this transformation with a greater vibrancy of body, mind, and spirit. I promise.

2.

Ann Louise's All-Star Peri Zappers

The Tried-and-True Method for Hormonal Harmony

Perimenopausal symptoms are many, but the primary causes are relatively few. Only rarely do two women have exactly the same symptoms, but their symptoms frequently share the same causes. However, symptoms and their origins often cannot be tied together in a direct cause-and-effect relationship.

The fundamental cause of perimenopausal symptoms is hormonal imbalance, chiefly that between progesterone and estrogen in the menstrual cycle. The two most important causes of hormonal imbalance are a lack of regular ovulation and an exhaustion of the adrenal glands.

Hormonal Imbalance

Estrogen and progesterone counter each other's effects. When their levels rise and fall, as they should in a normal menstrual cycle, they are in balance and you do not suffer from symptoms. At most, you may have minor discomfort or inconvenience on menstruation, but you do not have PMS or perimenopause symptoms at any time during the cycle.

When the estrogen-progesterone balance is disrupted, things go wrong. Eating a lot of processed carbohydrates and sugar causes an imbalance of estrogen and progesterone as well as of insulin. Poor eating habits and inadequate nutrition, resulting in vitamin or mineral deficiencies, also throws off estrogen and progesterone levels. So, too, do very low-fat diets, which deprive the body of the good fats it needs to stay healthy and manufacture hormones. Stress can also be a major problem, leaving its mark on the menstrual cycle. While women can go for years without showing any ill effects from an unhealthy lifestyle, poor nutrition, and high stress, the payoff is likely to be symptoms in their mid-thirties to late forties—the perimenopause years.

At some point during your perimenopause, you stop ovulating regularly. This can begin at any time from your mid-thirties to your late forties. You may skip an occasional month or go two or more successive months without ovulating. When no egg ripens in your ovaries, there is no empty follicle to turn into a corpus luteum and secrete progesterone. This is when you start having mood swings, weight gain, and water retention.

Even when no ovulation occurs and no progesterone is secreted, the menstrual cycle proceeds. Estrogen causes the uterine lining to be shed, and menstrual flow takes place—though it may be very light or irregular. Then the brain sends a message to the ovaries, and a new cycle begins. You may go several cycles on estrogen alone and experience estrogen dominance.

Some women have irregular periods for many years. They may notice light flow or only "spotting." Occasional heavy flows may signify ovulation and a return of progesterone. The fact that they are still menstruating causes many of these women to assume their symptoms have nothing to do with hormones. Some women have few or no symptoms, while the lives of others are made miserable. And there are many grades between these two extremes.

When a woman doesn't ovulate for many successive months, her

Symptoms Caused or Made Worse by Estrogen Dominance

Aging process accelerated	Headaches
Allergies	Hypoglycemia
Autoimmune disorders (for example, lupus)	Infertility
	Irritability
Blood clotting increase (raising risk of stroke)	Memory loss
	Miscarriage
Bone loss before menopause	Osteoporosis
Breast tenderness	PMS
Depression	Sex drive decrease
Fat gain (especially around abdomen, hips, thighs)	Thyroid dysfunction mimicking hypothyroidism
Fatigue	Uterine cancer
Fibrocystic breasts	Uterine fibroids
Foggy thinking	Water retention and bloating
Gallbladder disease	

ovaries' secretion of estrogen can become erratic. She may have surges of the hormone followed by unusually low levels. With estrogen surges, she is likely to suffer from water retention, weight gain, breast swelling and tenderness, sleep disturbance, and mood swings. But usually her estrogen levels remain normal, and the symptoms that she feels are caused mainly by her lack of progesterone.

If this woman has her hormone levels tested at a doctor's office, the physician typically will order lab tests for the estrogen estradiol and for the follicle-stimulating hormone (FSH) and luteinizing hormone (LH), both brain messengers to the ovaries. Only rarely will her progesterone level be measured. Depending on when in her cycle she is tested and on whether she is tested only once, which is typical, her estrogen level may appear low and her FSH high. In this event, the doctor may recommend that she take estrogen, which would be the last thing she needs in an already estrogen-dominant situation. Fortunately, the doctor is more likely to make a more benevolent misdiagnosis—that of emotional causes.

In remedying perimenopause symptoms, I take a holistic approach. By this, I mean that I don't approach symptoms as separate, independent entities, putting a patch on one here and another one there. Instead, I try to heal the underlying cause, by restoring the balance of the five interconnected hormonal systems: blood sugar, stress, sex, hunger, and antiaging. I do this through the Peri Prescription (detailed in chapter 15). With the Peri Prescription as an underlying stabilizing influence, I also use successive Peri Zappers (detailed later in this chapter) to cure perimenopause symptoms. I believe in starting out with the mildest remedy possible—that is, implementing the first three or four Peri Zappers.

The Peri Zappers are remedies based on my own personal experiences during perimenopause and on the experiences of thousands of women I have assisted over the years as a nutritionist. As you read on, you will meet the Zappers and see why they do the things they do. You will also meet a number of my clients in this and the following chapters. I will always be so grateful and thankful to all of these women and the many other clients who have shared with me so much by documenting their successful use of diet, nutrients, natural remedies, stress relief, and exercise.

Andrea

"I hate listening to people whine," Andrea said, sitting across my desk from me. "I hate listening to myself do it even more."

"People don't come here to tell me about the wonderful things in their lives," I assured her.

She asked if she could smoke, and I said no. Andrea sighed, put away the pack of cigarettes she had already opened, and said, "Look at my skin. Look how dry the skin on my arms is, and that's after I put on moisturizer only a couple of hours ago. Look at the wrinkles. Every day I see more of them. Look at my face. I'm forty-four. How old do I look to you?" She gazed at me with lackluster eyes. "I swear, every time I look in the mirror, I see myself visibly older than when I last looked at myself. It's like something out of a late-night horror movie."

"That's not necessarily aging, Andrea," I said. "Your skin may simply be reflecting a deficiency in your body. Fix that deficiency, and your skin can recover."

"It's not just my skin," she went on. "My whole body is breaking down, falling to pieces. My mind too. All at the same time! And I can't do anything about it!"

"I can—with your help," I volunteered.

"I hope so," she murmured, a hint of skepticism in her voice from so many false promises and demoralizing failed attempts. "Let me tell you the rest, and maybe you won't be so sure. I've become fifteen pounds overweight in less than two years. But if you'd seen me about ten days ago, I looked like I was thirty pounds overweight because I was so darn bloated. Then it went away. I don't understand why. Also, I've been getting the most terrible headaches recently, right across the front of my forehead. And I get depressed. God, do I get depressed! It's not just feeling sorry for myself because I'm falling to pieces. This depression hits me from nowhere—drops on me like a black cloud and presses down on me."

"I feel confident I can help you," I said, empathizing with Andrea's litany of symptoms and the distress they were causing her.

"There's one more thing," she warned. "I have no energy. I'm tired all the time. That's where I thought you could help, by giving me special vitamins and stuff that would at least get me up and going, so I could do something about all the other things, instead of sitting and staring into space."

"I can do better than that," I said, encouraged she had listed all of her symptoms instead of talking only about the fatigue. "Do you miss any periods?"

"Occasionally. Maybe twice a year."

We went on to talk about her lifestyle. Apart from cigarette smoking, frequent dieting was her main unhealthy pastime. When I told her that she didn't have a dozen different things wrong with her but only one—unbalanced hormones—she looked at me incredulously, eyebrows raised, eyes narrowed, and head cocked to the left. Nonetheless, she agreed to follow my instructions, giving me six weeks to produce results. She would do everything I said—except give up cigarettes.

I put her on the Peri Prescription to help stabilize her hormones. Knowing that the diet on its own might not be sufficient in her case, I also had her include more of Peri Zapper #1: flaxseeds and/or flax oil. After only two weeks, she reported that her skin definitely looked smoother. Now, if only I could do something about her general well-being . . . Although I usually recommend trying the Zappers in numerical order, I suggested that she skip to #5, natural progesterone cream, because this remedy is so all-encompassing, and this client wanted results yesterday. Nine or ten days later, she emailed to say that this was the magic potion she had been looking for. It was taking care of everything! Andrea paid me another visit a month later. She said she felt like the best version of herself. I happily watched her run her fingers through her hair as she told me about how much fuller it felt. Her once sad eyes now sparkled with hope.

She was in such a good mood, she even listened to what I had to say about smoking and promised to try a strategy I suggested. This involved gradually cutting back the number she smoked every day. If she could possibly cut down to five to ten per day, she would no longer have a powerful nicotine addiction. She would find it relatively easy to stop smoking by almost any method she chose.

More than a year later, Andrea was still struggling, but she was getting there. Thankfully, she had much less of a struggle with her perimenopause symptoms. The Peri Prescription, flaxseed oil, natural progesterone cream, and moderate exercise made the symptoms more or less disappear. She also found that B complex vitamins seem to smooth over the rough surfaces in her mind *and* her body.

Meet the Peri Zappers

As you meet the Peri Zappers in numerical order, you will read a short introduction to each member of this all-star team. There are no rookies here! All these Zappers are combat-hardened veterans from the perimenopause wars. Don't forget that they work best when you're on the Peri Prescription (see chapter 15).

Although the Zappers are presented in ascending order of strength, don't automatically assume that the strongest is the one you must try because of your severe symptoms. Time and time again, I have found the mildest Zappers work miracles, especially when taken in conjunction with the Peri Prescription, a powerful hormone balancer in and of itself.

#1 PERI ZAPPER
Flaxseeds and/or Flaxseed Oil

Flaxseeds and flaxseed oil contain both omega-3 and omega-6 fatty acids. Flax contains the parent oil or biochemical precursor of the fatty acids EPA (eicosapentaenoic acid) and DHA (docosahexaenoic acid), which transform into hormone-like prostaglandins. Because flax helps to balance estrogen, it is a great remedy for perimenopausal symptoms, especially skin conditions, depression, and fatigue. It also fights cancer (especially breast cancer), lowers cholesterol levels, and makes insulin more effective. And there's more! Flax discourages the body from storing fat, enhances the immune system, and reduces the risk of osteoporosis!

When using flaxseeds, make sure they are ground to release the nutrients. You can grind fresh flaxseeds in a coffee grinder kept especially for spices and sprinkle them on salads or cereals, or mix them into muffins. You can also buy flaxseeds that have been pre-ground, often available as flaxseed meal.

Please note that if you have thyroid conditions, you may wish to toast the flaxseeds yourself in an oven at 250°F for ten to fifteen minutes. This process deactivates and decomposes the cyanogenic glycosides while also maintaining the omega-3 properties. Cyanogenic glycosides metabolize into the chemical thiocyanate, which over time has the potential to suppress the thyroid's ability to take up sufficient iodine.

Flaxseed oil has a nutty flavor. People who don't care for this taste or for the consistency of the oil can swallow it quickly and wash it down with tea or some other drink. Because heat, light, and oxygen quickly cause the oil to become rancid, it should be purchased only in a black, opaque bottle, which should be refrigerated after being opened. Obviously, it should not be used in cooking or baking, although it can be poured on hot food. Take 1 or 2 tablespoons daily, as a salad dressing or drizzled over any side dish, such as a baked potato, steamed vegetable, or, my favorite, a popcorn snack.

#2

PERI ZAPPER

Black Currant Seed Oil

Black currant seed oil is a potent source of gamma-linolenic acid (GLA), a fatty acid that converts into hormone-like prostaglandins, which have a variety of functions, including stimulating fat burn. I believe GLA is a miracle ingredient, especially for cramping, irritability, headaches, and water retention. While there are several oils that contain GLA, I recommend black currant seed oil because it provides the most balanced form of omega-3 (alpha-linolenic acid) and omega-6 essential fatty acids.

To relieve breast tenderness, mood changes, anxiety, irritability, headaches, and water retention, take two capsules of 90 milligram GLA derived from black currant seed oil twice daily after food.

#3

PERI ZAPPER

M 'n' M (Magnesium and Multivitamins)

A combo of magnesium and certain vitamins may be necessary to get your hormonal systems back in balance. M 'n' M is a marvelous supplement mix for the mind as well as the body, helping to smooth out mood swings and combat fibromyalgia, panic attacks, insomnia, anxiety, tissue dryness, and water retention. Involved in more than 350 biochemical processes of the body, magnesium is notoriously deficient in most women in the perimenopausal stage of life. It works with vitamin B6 and zinc to alleviate a broad spectrum of perimenopause symptoms.

MAGNESIUM: 400 to 1,000 milligrams throughout the day. Generally you should take 5 milligrams of magnesium per pound of body weight, according to functional medicine experts.

VITAMIN B COMPLEX: should include 50 to 100 milligrams of activated vitamin B6, with at least 800 micrograms of methylated folate and at least 1,000 micrograms of methylated B12 taken once daily

VITAMIN C: 1,000 milligrams three times a day

VITAMIN E: 400 to 1,200 international units daily

When you feel that your hormones are back in better balance, you may be able to cut back to 1,000 milligrams a day of vitamin C and to 400 international units daily of vitamin E.

#4 PERI ZAPPER
Zinc

If M 'n' M doesn't completely clear up your symptoms, try a zinc supplement of 15 to 50 milligrams a day. This mineral is a must if you are vegetarian, as zinc is usually found in animal products. Zinc helps to lower estrogen and increase progesterone levels, build strong bones, and keep your immune system in tip-top shape to ward off viruses. It will also balance your copper levels. When your body transforms the levels of "free copper" to a bioavailable form, you may experience increased energy, less anxiety, and fewer mood swings.

#5 PERI ZAPPER
Natural Progesterone Cream

Perimenopausal symptoms are frequently caused by a low progesterone level. Taking an artificial progesterone (progestin) can intensify your symptoms and also make your body feel that something is not quite right. Natural progesterone is the same molecule as that in your body. Used as a non-prescription skin cream, it rebuilds your body's progesterone level, restores hormonal balance, and helps relieve a wide array of symptoms, including decreased sex drive, depression, abnormal blood sugar levels, fatigue, fuzzy thinking, irritability, thyroid dysfunction, water retention, bone loss, fat gain, and low adrenal function.

See details about choosing a high-quality natural progesterone cream and its proper application in chapter 7.

#6
PERI ZAPPER
The Right Moves

Exercise positively influences the sex hormones and supports the adrenals, reducing cortisol levels. Get up and moving at least five days a week. You can opt for half an hour of vigorous activity or try the shorter, but more intense, high-intensity interval training (HIIT). Or both! Either form will lower insulin resistance, reduce stress, balance hormones, and improve glucose tolerance, which, in turn, balances blood sugar. Do housework, garden, walk briskly, cycle, swim, dance, have fun. Do different things each day—and do what you enjoy! This Peri Zapper is especially important if you spend all day sitting down for work or have an otherwise sedentary lifestyle. Be sure not to over-exercise; keep strenuous activity to less than two continuous hours in order to avoid overstressing your body.

#7
PERI ZAPPER
Stress Reliever

Stress, while an essential survival response, can cause cortisol levels to go haywire, digestion to slow, depression and anxiety to set in, the brain to shrink, and a "menopot"—the belly fat that often appears during perimenopause—to develop. Lowering stress levels will also help to offset the aging process, which is accelerated by excess cortisol.

Top-notch stress relievers include brisk walking, deep breathing, and meditation. Please see all my suggestions on how to manage stress and keep your stress hormone cortisol in check in chapter 9.

#8
PERI ZAPPER
Adrenal Refresher

Adrenal recovery is very important during perimenopause. The adrenals are the backup system for the reproductive organs and are designed to make up for the declining hormone output. In order to perform this function, the adrenals need a full supply of vitamins, minerals, and adaptogens for optimized health.

In order to achieve this, consider Uni Key's Female Multiple and Uni Key's Adrenal Formula (see Resources), as well as adding pantethine to your program. Pantethine is the biologically active form of pantothenic acid, the stress vitamin. I typically like to see 1,000 milligrams twice per day.

#9 PERI ZAPPER
Liver and Bile Support

Support your liver so that it can produce enough quality bile, which is necessary to break down fats and transport excess hormones out of the body. Inadequate bile leads to poor estrogen metabolism, hypothyroidism, fatigue, indigestion, constipation, and weight gain. This will in turn provoke perimenopause-related symptoms.

To support the liver and produce quality bile, consider supplementing your morning smoothie with beet powder or taking bile salts (100 to 200 milligrams per meal) as well as adding 1 to 2 tablespoons of non-GMO soy or sunflower lecithin granules to soups or salads. The supplement Bile Builder (see Resources) contains all the nutrients known to decongest the liver and thin the bile—500 milligrams choline, 50 milligrams lipase, 250 milligrams taurine, 100 milligrams ox bile (extract or salt), 100 milligrams beet root, and 60 milligrams collinsonia root (to aid in breaking down stones). Studies have shown that foods such as eggs, onions, and pork are the top three gallbladder allergens, so avoiding these foods may help both the liver and bile function and flow smoothly.

#10 PERI ZAPPER
Natural Estrogen Therapy

You don't have to take horse estrogen and artificial progesterone (progestin), subjecting yourself to a risk of breast cancer and to weird bodily feelings. Instead, you can take the natural hormone estriol, specially prepared for your needs as indicated by saliva tests of your hormone levels. With your healthcare practitioner's help, you can determine the proper dose for your body's needs.

Taking phytoestrogens (plant estrogens) also can moderate your estrogen levels and ease your symptoms as you reach menopause. I recommend both foods and supplements of pomegranate seed oil, maca, curcumin, and a Thai vine called *Pueraria mirifica*. Please follow recommendations on the labels for the various seeds, tinctures, oils, and pills.

3.

Controlling Carbs

The Perimenopause Solution for Weight Gain, the Munchies, and a Short Attention Span

Surprisingly, depression, mood swings, and impaired cognitive function, such as a shortened memory or attention span, may have just as much to do with diet as with perimenopause itself. These symptoms often seem to go away when women switch to the Peri Prescription, which simultaneously balances blood sugar and hormone levels. So many clinical research studies associate depression and mood swings with hypoglycemia (low blood sugar) that we can confidently look to diet as the mainline therapy.

Fat, not sugar, is the body's primary fuel source—a concept that runs totally counter to the prevailing dietary dogma. That being said, carbohydrates are the body's best source of glucose, making carbs a key source of energy. Contrary to popular belief, carbohydrates are not only those notorious slices of bread and freshly baked cookies you hear vilified in popular diet rhetoric. One of the three macronutrients (along with protein and fat), carbohydrates actually encompass all the starches, fibers, and sugars found in grains, fruits, vegetables, beans, legumes, milk, and milk products.

So why, then, have carbs gotten such a bad reputation? Well, not all carbs are created equal—and it's not as simple as the difference between simple and complex carbohydrates. What matters is where the carbs come from. Different sources of carbohydrates have different impacts on blood sugar levels. Carbs from low-sugar, *unprocessed*, plant-based sources (like vegetables and beans) take longer to digest, so they can provide the body with all the good nutrients that carbs have to offer while not causing dramatic changes in blood sugar levels. Carbs from high-sugar, *processed* sources (think desserts and any foods made with grains that have been ground into flour) are digested quickly, creating erratic changes in the body's blood sugar levels. Unbalanced blood sugar levels have significant, unwanted impacts on your health, disrupting hormones and exacerbating perimenopause symptoms, such as increased fat storage and mood swings.

This description is only a generalization, and the difference between "good" and "bad" carbohydrates is more complex. But as you read this chapter, you will learn how to think through this carb conundrum and use carbohydrates as a tool in navigating hormonal health.

The Sugar Swing

When you eat a less than ideal carbohydrate, your blood sugar level quickly soars, followed by a quick and unpleasant crash landing. As your blood sugar drops, your brain becomes frantic for its only source of fuel—glucose—and that's when sugar cravings and bingeing begin. During the low blood sugar period, you can feel mood swings, irritability, and a lack of attention, and even undergo a weight shift. This roller-coaster ride of high and low blood sugar is caused by hormones reacting to the food you have eaten—primarily reactions between carbohydrates and the pancreatic hormone insulin, between proteins and the pancreatic hormone glucagon, and between fats and the hormones called eicosanoids. A fundamental solution to your symptoms, whether they are related to blood sugar or perimenopause, is an eating plan that consists of high-quality, unprocessed carbohydrates along with high-quality fats and proteins that keep insulin levels low and help to stabilize blood sugar levels.

Most women—particularly when in the perimenopause stage, from the late twenties to the late forties—have been brainwashed about the benefits of a low-fat, high-complex-carbohydrate diet plan. This unbalanced eating regimen has created many of the symptoms we now attribute to perimenopause.

For as long as I can remember, I have been warning about the dangers of fat-free, carb-rich diets. When I was director of nutrition at the Pritikin Longevity Center in Santa Monica in the early 1980s, I first noticed that many people on a diet low in fat and high in complex carbohydrates often suffered from low energy, fatigue, mood swings, allergies, yeast infections, and dry skin, hair, and nails. I wrote about the struggles of these individuals in my first book, *Beyond Pritikin*. I believe the symptoms I saw many people experience were diet based, caused by a lack of essential fatty acids that we normally get in the "good" dietary fats and an overemphasis on carbohydrates from such reactive grains as wheat. Science is now proving my hypothesis to be true. (We will take a deeper dive into the satisfying and special contributions of sexy, slimming fats in the next chapter.)

When you cut these smart fats from your diet, you are likely to develop food cravings and go on eating binges. Your body will "beg" you to make up for the missing fats by craving large amounts of carbohydrates, such as bread, muffins, bagels, fat-free cookies, and low-fat yogurt.

Today, large numbers of otherwise careful eaters don't realize that many of the complex carbohydrates they eat act in the same way as processed simple carbohydrates by causing a surge in their blood sugar levels. They have a basic misunderstanding about the difference between good and bad carbohydrates, as does much of mainstream society in the United States. Ironically, some of those highly touted and commonly consumed complex carbohydrates, like whole-grain bread and other grain-based foods, can create the same blood sugar peaks and valleys as sweets. You see, even whole-grain flour is still a processed version of carbohydrates. I cannot imagine how many health-conscious people are frustrated with their body for craving a high-sugar snack or soft drink when, in reality, their diet has created a biological sugar trap masquerading as a "lack of willpower."

Heather

An accountant for a chain of stores, Heather put in many sedentary hours at her work. But she made up for it in her free time, she told me. At forty-one, she walked briskly a few miles with her husband every day, rain or shine, year-round. However, she expressed her frustr to me that, despite her physical activity, she was still about fifteen pounds overweight. I noticed Heather's manner was at first outgoing and charming, but then she seemed to lapse into a sort of tiredness, even despondency, after only a few minutes of conversation with me.

"I can't lose weight, no matter what I try," she told me. "Every time I relax my vigilance with food, I put on another pound, which of course I then can't lose. So I went to a dietitian. She put me on a low-fat diet and had me getting 55 percent of my calories from carbs, 20 percent from protein, and 25 percent from fats. You know what happened? I began to feel tired all the time. So I stopped seeing the dietitian."

"And then what happened?" I prompted her.

She sighed. "I tried other low-fat diets, but I kept noticing my moodiness getting worse, and I had a hard time getting my work done. Nowadays I am always getting distracted. Scrolling through Facebook or talking to my friends just seems more interesting than being productive, especially when I can't even focus on my spreadsheets in the first place. To tell you the truth, I am beginning to wonder if I am suffering from attention deficit disorder, especially after talking to some of the other moms whose children had been diagnosed. I can't stop my mind from wandering. This has been going on now for more than a year, and I can feel that I'm getting worse. I started out being worried about my weight. Weight is the least of my worries now. I'm an accountant, and I can't concentrate!"

I sympathized with her, having had numerous clients with similar experiences. When I asked what she ate on a typical day, she gave me the following thumbnail sketch of her eating habits:

BREAKFAST: a cup of coffee with almond milk and cold cereal with a sliced banana

MIDMORNING: to combat tiredness, an energy bar and grapes

LUNCH: a side salad and a chicken wrap with spinach, shredded cheese, and ranch dressing

MIDAFTERNOON: a low-fat yogurt as a pick-me-up

DINNER: lots of veggies and a handful of shrimp stir-fried in a nonstick pan (using no oil), with lots of brown rice

AFTER DINNER: feeling famished, frequent trips to the refrigerator for fat-free ice cream, frozen yogurt, cookies, and more fruit

I pointed out to her that basically all she was eating was sugar, sugar, sugar. Even the complex carbs—for example, brown rice at dinner—were fast acting or high-glycemic. I finally talked her into an egg for breakfast or some organic peanut butter on an apple wedge as she was flying out the door. For lunch, she needed poultry, tuna, or seafood without cheese and heavy dressing. At midafternoon, some almonds. For a basic dinner, I suggested salad, lean beef or tofu, green vegetables, and a small sweet potato. I pleaded with her to put a couple of teaspoons of extra-virgin olive oil on her salads, and to eat nuts.

"Just watch your carbs," I warned her.

In eyeballing her portions, she needed to recognize that an average-size portion of chicken, beef, or fish was about the size of a deck of cards. A serving of vegetables and starchy food, such as pasta, potatoes, or corn, should be no bigger than a tennis ball. In this serving, ideally there should be three times as much vegetable as starchy food. A teaspoon of oil is about the size of a quarter.

With a little practice, visual estimates of serving sizes become easy and almost second nature. They are of great value in eating out, when you can ease excess quantities to one side of your plate and avoid overeating or unbalanced eating. A food that is fat-free, like pasta or rice, needs to be portion controlled because the insulin response can prompt the body to store excess calories as body fat.

In less than a week, Heather had made a total diet transition. That was all the time it took on her new diet to break the habit of nighttime refrigerator visits. In less than a month, she noticed the difference in her powers of concentration at work. She began to feel better in her body. Over time, she felt more balanced emotionally and physically, and had the energy to make it through a session with me without yawning. She lost weight and felt fitter, finding it easy to stick to a diet that made her mind and body function better than they ever had. Heather had finally listened to her body, responding to its cries for proper fuel by eating a more nutritious, high-fat, low-carb diet—exactly what it wanted.

Heather continued to do well. When I last saw her, she was bubbly and bright as well as trim and active. It had been a long time since she had last felt tired, moody, or depressed. Give the body what it needs, and you shall receive!

Carbohydrates and Blood Sugar

Your body has two critical reactions when you eat carbohydrates. First, it converts all carbohydrates into blood sugar in the form of glucose. Second, it releases insulin. Insulin is a hormone secreted by the pancreas that regulates glucose levels in the blood. It metabolizes blood sugar so that muscle tissue can use it for fuel, and it also helps store excess blood sugar, either in the liver or tissues as glycogen or elsewhere in the body as fat.

In a balanced state, our bloodstream contains about 2 teaspoons of glucose. The carbohydrates that we eat easily supply this amount of glucose—and all too easily exceed the amount we need. The blood sugar that our bodies do not use as fuel is stored as body fat, under the control of insulin. With our bodies' blood sugar requirements so easily met, the last thing we need to eat is processed carbohydrates (flour, pasta, white rice) or excessive amounts of potatoes, corn chips, or brown rice. All these carbohydrates rapidly convert into glucose and cause a sharp rise in our blood sugar level, resulting in a sharp rise in our insulin level, which then stores excess blood sugar as body fat. This is why people who eat a lot of low-fat pasta dishes can actually put on weight instead of losing it!

The last thing women in perimenopause need is another force in their bodies, like excess blood sugar, destabilizing their hormones. As you now know, carbohydrate-induced blood sugar swings can cause disrupted mood, lack of concentration, fatigue, weight gain, and more. During perimenopause, the body is going through enough hormonal gymnastics already; no need to get on a blood sugar roller coaster too.

At this point some women will throw up their hands in despair. What are they to do? The first step is simply to accept the following two facts: First, there are good and bad dietary fats, and our bodies need the good ones. Good dietary fats are actually the body's best blood sugar stabilizer. Second, the food we eat evokes hormonal responses in our bodies. The next step is to move away from a low-fat diet of 55 percent carbohydrates, 20 percent protein, and 25 percent (or less) fats, and toward a hormone-regulating diet of 40 percent fats, 30 percent carbs, and 30 percent protein. Of course, these percentages are approximate proportions for the three macronutrients and should not be strictly interpreted.

Telling the smart fats from the dumb fats is easy, as you will see in the next chapter. It's not as easy to get familiar with the different types of carbohydrate foods. Which of them evoke rapid blood sugar and insulin responses? Which are digested more slowly and therefore evoke a less steep rise in blood sugar and, consequently, a less steep rise in the fat storage hormone insulin? Read on to become your own carbohydrate detective, and learn how to investigate labels and ingredients to find the best carbs for your body.

The Good News!

Your body needs carbohydrates. It needs the right ones at the right time. Vegetables, beans, and nuts are just a few of the delicious carbohydrates that can inundate your body with necessary energy and health benefits. These good carbohydrates are excellent sources of fiber. Fiber not only keeps your digestive system functioning regularly but also lowers blood pressure, supports intestinal flora, and has numerous other benefits, upon which I will expound later in this chapter. Good carbohydrates also support adrenal function by helping to stabilize cortisol levels, leading to decreased stress, improved sleep, and overall improved body function.

Let's explore how a smart approach to eating carbs can support your transition through perimenopause.

First, I want you to watch your high sugar and/or processed carb intake to start to improve sugar-related hormone imbalances and the difficult symptoms they cause. But reduce your intake slowly to protect your hormone production and metabolism, and reduce cravings. If you eliminate the sugars and high-glycemic foods gradually, you will not suffer too much from symptoms of sugar detoxification.

At the same time, you must increase your intake of sexy, slimming fats, eat more vegetables, and enjoy healthful proteins. If you eat meat, please consume animals raised on pastures. There are a myriad of reasons for this, which I will discuss later, but know that factory-farmed, grain-fed meat is particularly disruptive to your hormones.

You will know if you are consuming the right balance of carbs to properly support your hormones by your energy level, mood, brain function, and quality of sleep. If these seem to be suffering, please add a bit more healthful carbs to your diet. If you are gaining weight or experiencing other symptoms of carbohydrate overload that I have described in this chapter, eat fewer carbs. Keep a journal to monitor your reactions to different foods and the amount of carbohydrates. This will allow you to clearly see where on the carb teeter-totter you need to sit.

A study at the Hebrew University of Jerusalem found that eating carbs at dinner may be the most beneficial. The study showed that consuming carbohydrates at dinner resulted in increased weight loss, improved blood sugar, a reduction in inflammation, and other benefits to the metabolism when compared to participants who spread their carb consumption throughout the day. Participants also experienced improved leptin, ghrelin, and adiponectin levels—three hormones that affect appetite, satiation, and fat burning (see chapter 4).

The Bad News . . .

If you are going to eat a carbohydrate, it probably should not be a grain, and it definitely should not be wheat. Health experts like neurologist Dr. David Perlmutter and cardiologist Dr. William Davis believe the consumption of wheat and other grains contributes to a substantial amount of illness, obesity, and suffering in humans today. Virtually all disease involves some kind of inflammation, and consuming grains like wheat causes inflammation, not only in the digestive system but throughout the body. As a matter of fact, in his book *Brain Maker,* Dr. Perlmutter implicates grain consumption as a major player in Alzheimer's and dementia, depression, attention deficit hyperactivity disorder (ADHD), digestive disorders like Crohn's disease, celiac disease, and irritable bowel syndrome (IBS), and many more, largely due to its inflammatory effects.

All grains have storage proteins called prolamins, but gluten—a protein composite found in wheat, rye, barley, and triticale—is known to be especially inflammatory and irritating to the immune system, and particularly difficult for the body to digest. Reactions to gluten are even worse for those with a genetic susceptibly to celiac disease and gluten sensitivity. Studies have shown that gluten activates a protein in the digestive tract called zonulin, which regulates the opening of spaces between cells in the intestinal lining that allow molecules to flow in and out. This overactivation of zonulin creates increased intestinal permeability, also known as leaky gut syndrome, leading to inflammation in the gut. Leaky gut syndrome is linked to an increase in a range of devastating health conditions, including autoimmunity, diabetes, and cancer. The expansive effects of gluten may even influence brain and behavior, with gluten-induced inflammation possibly triggering mood disruptions like depression.

In addition, gliadin—the prolamin found in wheat gluten—is considered an opiate; it binds to the opiate receptors in the brain, stimulating appetite. It is both inflammatory and addictive. Gliadin also resembles thyroid hormone and can disrupt normal thyroid functioning (see chapter 10).

One more bit of bad news: As Dr. Davis points out in his book *Wheat Belly,* the wheat grain available today has less nutritional value than the wheat grown and consumed by our ancestors. Most whole-wheat products are now made from a wheat grain that was hybridized in the 1960s and 1970s, and modern wheat breads contain ten times as much gluten compared to breads made before the grain with gliadin was hybridized. Experts—like Dr. Alessio Fasano, who authored more than two hundred studies on the matter—now believe that our bodies simply cannot fully digest gluten, let alone the amount contained in modern wheat. Plus, much of today's gluten-rich grains are grown using Roundup, an herbicide produced by Monsanto that contains glyphosate. Glyphosate has been linked to cancer, a decrease in progesterone production, antibiotic resistance, and birth defects in rats.

A decade ago most of us had never even heard of gluten. Today many health-conscious consumers are trying to avoid it. I say that is an excellent idea. And while you're at it, why not avoid the rest of the wheat too.

Insulin Resistance and Other Disorders

The human insulin system evolved over thousands of years to process nutrients from natural, unprocessed foods, which it does with exceeding efficiency. But insulin has not yet had time to adapt to nutrients from modern foods, particularly the large amount of carbohydrates from grains. Until humans became agrarian, which took place comparatively late in our development, carbohydrates from grains were only a small part of our diet.

Frequent alternation of blood sugar/insulin highs and lows from eating too many bad, processed carbohydrates is thought to cause insulin resistance after prolonged exposure. The body becomes progressively less sensitive to insulin, and increasing amounts of the hormone are required to process the glucose. Insulin resistance is believed to be responsible when, as in many cases, overweight people cannot lose weight on a low-fat, high-carbohydrate diet.

In its most extreme form, insulin resistance can develop into type 2 diabetes. Diabetes develops when the pancreas cannot produce enough insulin, creating a shortage, or when the insulin is no longer effective in getting blood sugar into the muscle cells. As a result, the body can't metabolize the glucose, getting less of it for energy, which only causes more blood sugar to be stored as fat. Nerve and muscle cells become lethargic in the process as they are robbed of their main energy source.

According to the CDC, more than twenty-nine million people in the United States—nearly 10 percent of the country's population—are thought to have type 2 diabetes, and more than a quarter of them are undiagnosed. The American Heart Association reports that a person with type 2 diabetes is two to four times more likely to get cardiovascular disease. Even worse, nearly one in three people in the United States has prediabetes, according to the CDC, which is when blood sugar is higher than normal, and most of them don't know it!

Type 2 diabetes affects twice as many women as men over the age of forty-five. In cases of obesity-related type 2 diabetes, weight loss alone can be enough to control or cure the condition. Perimenopause is certainly the time when a woman needs to check whether her diet regulates her blood sugar hormones as she prepares herself for substantial hormonal changes. Getting these hormones in balance now with the Peri Prescription does much to ensure good health in future years.

If you think you might be diabetic or prediabetic, visit your doctor for a blood test of your blood sugar (glucose) levels while fasting. A second test while fasting at a different time on another day is good for a comparison measurement. Normal glucose numbers vary throughout the day, but for a person without diabetes, a fasting blood sugar—meaning you have consumed no food for eight hours—should be under 100 mg/dL (milligrams of glucose per deciliter of blood). Before a meal, blood sugar should be between 70 and 99 mg/dL. After meals, blood sugar should be less than 140 mg/dL.

Type 2 diabetes generally forms part of the "metabolic syndrome," which is characterized by insulin resistance, obesity, and a range of cardiovascular risk factors, including high blood pressure, high triglycerides, and high cholesterol levels. If you have even one of the conditions combined with insulin resistance, you have metabolic syndrome.

Who gets metabolic syndrome, and why? According to a study published in the *Journal of the American Medical Association,* metabolic syndrome is thought to affect 35 percent of all U.S. adults and 50 percent of U.S. adults aged sixty or older. The condition develops over time, mainly due to a diet high in refined carbohydrates (such as sweets, breads, and flour/sugar-based snack foods that cause high insulin levels) and can eventually lead to insulin resistance and related disorders. Chronically high insulin promotes "spare tire" fat storage, raises blood pressure, and worsens blood fat profiles.

Studies have shown that women undergoing the changes during perimenopause and menopause carry a special risk for developing metabolic syndrome. A five-year-long Australian study tracked 265 women, aged forty-six to fifty-seven, as they progressed through menopause. The study found that a surprisingly high percentage of these women—nearly one in six—developed impaired fasting glucose levels. Researchers also have found that women with breast cancer and high levels of insulin were eight times more likely to develop a recurrence and die of the disease than were women who had normal insulin levels; and women with metabolic syndrome symptoms may be ten times more likely to die of colon cancer than women who did not have those symptoms.

People with metabolic syndrome need to be especially careful to avoid alcohol, sugar, and white flour. Getting regular exercise and losing weight are confirmed methods for improving insulin resistance.

As we gain increasing knowledge of hormones, we are likely to get a better understanding of the symptoms that many disorders share with perimenopause. In the meantime, it is enough to know that diet, hormones, and the presence or absence of many female symptoms are all interconnected. It may be many years before researchers work out all the intricate and marvelous interactions of blood sugar, stress, sex, hunger, and antiaging hormones—and how these interactions differ from woman to woman, but I'm convinced that one day we will know all this. My strategy in the Peri Prescription has been to take as broad an approach as possible to regulating hormones through nutrition and not to quibble over fine points that may be regarded as irrelevant in a year.

Honey, You Can Keep Your Sugar

Sweet in the mouth, but sour in the gut, too much sugar, especially refined (processed) sugar, sends your body into hormonal havoc. As you have read, continually exceeding your body's sugar needs causes your pancreas to secrete more insulin to handle the increase in blood sugar, eventually storing the extra sugar as fat. So just avoid the sugary foods like candy bars, right? Not quite.

Sugar is more than the white crystals you stir into your coffee. It masks itself insidiously in different foods. When a grain is ground into flour, it behaves exactly like sugar in the body. Just two slices of whole-wheat bread, high in amylopectin A—a sugar-spiking carb—can raise blood sugar levels higher than most candy bars!

Furthermore, many fruits contain high levels of fructose. Previously thought of as a "better" sugar because it does not trigger insulin release, fructose still has detrimental effects. Instead of insulin metabolizing fructose, fructose goes straight to the liver, the only organ that cannot metabolize it. The liver turns the fructose into triglycerides (a form of fat), which can eventually turn into another source of excess body fat and weight gain. High triglyceride levels are associated with heart disease, especially in women, and nonalcoholic fatty liver disease, of which there have been a skyrocketing number of cases.

Some especially high-fructose fruits are apples, mangoes, pears, and watermelons as well as dried fruits and fruit juices. Fructose is also found in other sweeteners, like agave nectar, honey, molasses, and the highly processed high-fructose corn syrup, as well as common flavor products like ketchup and balsamic vinegar.

Additionally, eating too much fructose, and sugar in general, can affect the proteins in your body. In excess, sugar cross-links with proteins in a process called glycation. Glycation results in advanced glycation end product, which makes tissues brittle and causes the irreversible breakdown of connective tissue. Brittle tissue creates wrinkly, saggy skin and cellulite. A 2014 study conducted at the University of Florida showed that drinking large quantities of soda, which contains high-fructose corn syrup, may play a role in cell aging.

Too much fruit also encourages the growth of yeast. If you have a yeast problem, avoid all fruits for at least ten days, or eat no more than one low-sugar piece of fruit a day.

What's Left?

Despair not! Not all fruits and grains harm your body. There are several nutritious, delicious grain-like seeds you can use as alternatives to wheat that will satisfy your body's carbohydrate requirements as well as enliven your meals. Millet, amaranth, buckwheat, and quinoa are all fantastic options for you to explore.

- MILLET is a gluten-free seed grain. It is nutrient- and antioxidant-rich, with magnesium, B vitamins, calcium, manganese, phosphorus, and tryptophan. The fiber will nourish your gut too.

- AMARANTH is a high-protein seed that will satisfy your desire for grains. It offers quality fiber and is higher in calcium, iron, phosphorous, and carotenoids than most vegetables. And, of course, it's gluten-free.

- BUCKWHEAT is another seed that is high in protein and fiber, and it's gluten-free. Buckwheat seeds are usually called "groats." Buckwheat is so rich in nutrients and antioxidants that it might be considered a "superfood." Made from the ground seeds, buckwheat flour also makes a mean pancake.

- QUINOA is a gluten-free grain that has become quite popular and is easily available in most supermarkets. It's the only grain source of protein recognized as complete, with all the essential amino acids needed for growth and development.

In addition, there are low-fructose fruits you can eat without fear of your blood sugar spiking. Blackberries, strawberries, raspberries, and wild blueberries are low in fructose, high in fiber, and chock-full of a type of antioxidant known as polyphenol, which helps break down fat and interferes with the production of new fat cells. Some other low-fructose fruits include

Apricot	Nectarine
Avocado	Orange
Blackberries	Papaya
Blueberries	Passionfruit
Cantaloupe	Peach
Cherries	Pineapple
Grapefruit	Plum
Honeydew melon	Raspberries
Kiwifruit	Rhubarb
Lemon	Strawberries
Lime	Tangelo
Mandarin	

Fiber

Fiber—or "roughage," as my grandmother used to say—is a type of indigestible carbohydrate that the body cannot turn into sugar. It aids in detoxification by helping the digestive system to remove waste, keeping the things you don't need moving and grooving all the way out of your body. When you do not get enough fiber, bile and stool—full of toxins your body wants to excrete—remain in your intestines for too long, and toxins can be reabsorbed back into the body. This good carbohydrate has a plethora of other health benefits, such as decreasing inflammation, lowering blood pressure, reducing cortisol levels, improving your cholesterol profile, and feeding healthy gut bacteria.

Fiber is not simply indigestible husks and skins. There are some partially digestible types of fiber, and our bodies need them all, digestible and indigestible, to stay in good health. Cellulose is the indigestible kind of fiber in nearly all vegetables and fruits; this is usually what we mean when we say "fiber." But we shouldn't ignore the other kinds of fiber, mixed with cellulose, that the human digestive system can partially break down. These include lignans, pectins, gums, and hemicelluloses. You can find all the types of fiber in unprocessed plant foods, like avocados, blackberries, blueberries, carrots, celery, chia seeds (the world's most fiber-rich food), coconut, flaxseeds (high in lignans), green leafy vegetables, jicama, oatmeal, peas, sweet potatoes, and squash.

Dietary fiber is known to lower estrogen dominance, a condition suffered by many women during perimenopause (see chapter 7). Studies show that women who stick to a high-fiber eating regimen have lower levels of estrogen in the bloodstream. Fiber binds to excess estrogens and helps to eliminate them from the body, excreting them in the bowel. Furthermore, estrogen is one of those substances that can be reabsorbed back into the body if stool or bile remains in the digestive system for too long. Fiber's famous poop-promoting properties increase digestive regularity and, in turn, decrease estrogen's opportunity to be reabsorbed into the body. A study by David P. Rose, reported in the *American Journal of Clinical Nutrition,* found that two months on a high-fiber diet reduced levels of estrone, the less desirable form of estrogen, without affecting the levels of either progesterone or estriol, the more desirable form of estrogen.

Impressed yet? Well, it gets better. Fiber has also been acknowledged as a fighter of cancer by helping to remove potentially dangerous substances from the intestines. Similarly, this beneficial carbohydrate has been in the limelight as a regulator of blood sugar hormones. Fiber slows the absorption of sugar and prevents surges in the levels of blood sugar and insulin. And the cherry on top: increasing dietary fiber is the number one predictor of long-term weight loss. Fiber makes you feel full and satisfied because it takes longer to digest, helping you to avoid unhealthy cravings and unintentional overeating. It also takes longer to chew fibrous foods, giving your body time to signal to your brain that it is becoming full and satiated. This gives you a chance to feel when your body is actually full.

As you have seen, the kinds and amounts of carbohydrates you eat are of prime importance in a hormone-regulating diet. Desirable high-fiber foods on the Peri Prescription include moderate and low-glycemic complex carbohydrates, such as chickpeas, black beans, lentils, yams, fruits, vegetables, and other unprocessed plant foods listed earlier.

4.

Sexy, Slimming Fats and Hormone-Friendly Proteins

Improving Weight, Sleep, Memory, Skin, and Hair

Since the mid-twentieth century, popular diet advice has heralded protein as a super nutrient while relegating fat to a dark corner, accusing it of all sorts of nasty health transgressions, such as weight gain and heart disease. But I believe protein has some major competition as the premier weight-stabilizing, hormone-balancing nutritional cornerstone—and this competition comes from none other than fat itself.

This is not to minimize the importance of protein. Protein is essential, especially to women trying to balance their hormones during perimenopause. If your body does not get enough protein from the food you eat, its ability to make new hormones, antibodies, and tissue slows down, and it may even break down existing body protein—such as muscle tissue—to supply its needs. If that starts to happen, your metabolism slows down further, and you burn fewer calories and fat. This is how a diet too high in carbohydrates and low in protein can cause a loss of muscle tone. Other symptoms resulting from too little protein in the diet include thinning skin, brittle nails, hair loss, food cravings, loss of sexual desire, fatigue, irritability, and mental confusion.

Nonetheless, most people have heard the praises sung of protein for weight loss and overall health, but when it comes to the "fat makes you fat" mantra of the past few decades, nothing could be further from the truth. It's a mantra I have been refuting for a very long time. In fact, when I wrote the first edition of my book *Eat Fat, Lose Weight* in 1999, I was the only nutritionist in the country to write about the importance of eating the right dietary fats.

The U.S. public has been brainwashed with a big fat lie—retold for well over fifty years. What's more, this lie covered all fats, not just the trans, hydrogenated, overly refined, and genetically modified commercial vegetable oils that actually will harm you. I'm talking sunflower, safflower, cottonseed, soybean, canola, and corn oils, which really aren't even vegetable oils. Yes, they are "plant-based" oils, but they are extracted from grains and seeds, not vegetables.

Truth be told, our fear of fats only began in the 1950s, thanks to the work of research scientist Ancel Keys, Ph.D., who conducted the Seven Countries Study in which he cherry-picked data to support his theory that fat consumption led to cardiovascular disease. Although considered "pioneering" back in the day, the study was deeply flawed. Yet the media ran with it, and by 1961 the American Heart Association, where Keys served on the nutritional advisory board, issued its first anti-fat guidelines. This resulted in the launching of the no- to low-fat diet dictum that—to this day—many health experts still recommend and rely upon as gospel.

However, many years of research by the National Institutes of Health, costing several hundred million dollars, failed to demonstrate a connection between eating fat and getting heart disease. So if you've spent years being afraid of fat, take a deep breath, because this chapter is about to show you there is no bogeyman in that fat closet. In reality, it's the critical combination of protein and fat that is absolutely foundational to stabilize perimenopause symptoms and your overall health.

Jessica

A client called to say that a close friend would be contacting me for an appointment. Hardly five minutes later, the phone rang. Jessica sounded overwrought and begged to see me immediately on an emergency basis. I gently raised the possibility of her visiting a hospital emergency clinic, but she told me it wasn't "that kind" of emergency. I agreed to add her at the end of an already overcrowded day's schedule.

When Jessica walked into my office, she looked so forlorn I was glad I'd worked her in. She quickly but gracefully plopped in the chair across from me and let out a loud sigh of exasperation. "I'm thirty-eight years old, and I look like I'm eighty!" she proclaimed more loudly than I expected.

Jessica went on, obviously worked up, to relay her concerns about her dull hair and dry, prematurely wrinkled skin. She said the inexplicable and unexpected changes to her body had bothered her for some time now, but her tipping point had come when her mother-in-law had taken notice of it on a recent visit.

"My mother-in-law came to stay with us for a few days," she told me. "We hadn't seen her for a couple of years. She has a tendency to be overly direct and say whatever is on her mind, so my husband and two kids kept out of her way as much as they could. I wish I could have too. I told myself that I wouldn't let her get under my skin this time, but of course she sniffed out my insecurities and dug in. She was hardly in the house an hour before she let loose. She first asked if anything was wrong. She then went on to say that she asks because it looks like I've aged ten years since she saw me last."

I understood Jessica's concern. Not only did she not understand the changes in her own body, but also it was obvious she was a perfectionist. Just in my first few minutes with her, Jessica had paused repeatedly to fix her hair and clothing, and corrected any grammar mistakes she had made in conversation. She wanted to present her best self, and invested a lot into feeling and looking as good as possible. I could see how deeply her mother-in-law's blunt comments must have hurt Jessica.

"She kept harping on and on about my looks and how old I look for my age," Jessica continued, becoming visibly more upset as she recalled events. "It was one thing for me to be upset with my body, but to hear someone else say it? A nightmare—especially from my mother-in-law. I could hardly wait to drive her to the airport yesterday morning. We got there nearly three hours before her plane took off, and I just left her there and sped away as quickly as I could."

She mentioned her friend's name. "She started with me at the diet clinic but dropped out after only a couple of weeks," Jessica said. "She told me that was when she started coming to see you. I had coffee with her this morning and told her about the things my mother-in-law had been saying and how much I hate what is happening with my body. That was when she compared her neck and hands to mine. She didn't have to say anything else. I asked for your phone number."

"That was the emergency?"

"You bet." She gave me a small smile. "Can you help?"

I smiled back, trying to reassure her. I was just happy she had come to me because I knew exactly how to help her.

Jessica told me she was rigorously following an extremely low-fat diet with which I was familiar. Some of its adherents, including Jessica, regarded all fat in food as more or less toxic. As a result of this over-zealousness, their bodies had lower than healthy levels of certain fatty acids that the body does not make itself. These fatty acids, called essential fatty acids, are necessary for the body's manufacture of important molecules that are the building blocks of hormones and other substances. In trying to avoid all fats, Jessica had likely deprived herself of even the good ones.

But could I be certain that her very-low-fat diet was the cause of her skin and hair problems? No, I could not. She had recently had a thorough physical, and no medical disorder had been diagnosed. So I ruled out that as a cause. What about perimenopause? She was thirty-eight, so it was possible.

The diet I put her on provided all the nutrients that her body required and regulated her blood sugar and other hormones. When she started to look better, she would worry less about her appearance, producing fewer stress hormones. My guess was that with her blood sugar and stress hormones in balance, she would not suffer symptoms from her ovarian hormones. But we would have to wait and see.

Jessica didn't see the improvement she wanted. It took a while for me to find out why. She finally admitted that she wasn't following my diet. She just couldn't bring herself to eat food that she knew contained fat. Jessica, like so many women her age, had been brainwashed by the previous generation to view fat as the ultimate dietary demon. After several attempts, I finally convinced her that Mediterranean women have been known to have the very best skin and hair I have ever seen. And all they used was extra-virgin olive oil in cooking and on salads. Finally, the turning point was when her acquaintances began remarking on how much better she was looking, after she had grudgingly agreed to add olive oil to her salad dressing. I needed to say no more! Jessica was now well on her way to recovering her youthful skin and hair.

Sexy, Slimming Fats? You Bet.

For the more than half a century that fat has been terribly maligned and misunderstood in the U.S. diet landscape, our health and waistlines have suffered for it. Other people around the world did not have this same lapse in scientific judgment about diet, and they have enjoyed superior health to that of many in the United States as a reward for their acuity. Italians and Greeks have been eating much the same diet, with high amounts of monounsaturated fat in the form of olive oil, for more than three thousand years. Their cardiovascular health is much better than ours, as is that of the French, who eat food rich in saturated fat (butter, cream, and liver pâtés) along with red wine. Despite earlier reports, people in countries that use a lot of palm oil and coconut oil, both rich in saturated fat, don't have high rates of cardiovascular disease. And how do the Maasai and some Eskimo live almost exclusively on saturated fat? Denouncing saturated fat as a public enemy is the easy way out. Study after study is proving fat's irreplaceable role in our health.

So what's so great about fat? Everything.

Fats are your best, most potent source of energy—not carbohydrates. Good fats give your body fuel without causing substantial changes in blood sugar levels like carbohydrates can. Because blood sugar levels remain steady when you eat fat, less insulin is released into the bloodstream, meaning less sugar is ultimately stored as fat and you experience fewer hormonal upsets. This also means that your body won't develop insulin resistance from continual insulin inundation, helping to prevent conditions like metabolic syndrome and type 2 diabetes.

Good fats also improve hunger hormone function in the body. Take leptin, for example. Leptin is secreted by body fat cells and tells your body whether it needs to pack on or shed pounds based on the amount of fat it is carrying. Good fat allows leptin to clearly communicate to your body whether to eat more or less in order to gain or lose weight. In the absence of good fat, that communication can get muddled. Like insulin, you can develop leptin resistance by eating too many refined carbs. When leptin resistant, the body is no longer sensitive to the appetite-decreasing effects of leptin, and you gain weight.

Another hunger hormone produced by fat cells in the body is adiponectin. It has been referred to as the body's "fat burning torch," and it spends its time circulating in the bloodstream. The more you have of adiponectin, the more fat you will burn for fuel, especially from the abdominal area. Low levels of adiponectin have been linked with higher levels of obesity and insulin resistance. How do you boost adiponectin levels? Well, with good fats, of course.

In addition, fats release the hormone cholecystokinin (CCK). CCK triggers an immediate feeling of fullness during a meal, sending a message to your brain that you are no longer hungry. Without this hormone, you will continue to feel hungry and dissatisfied after a meal. This explains why people who eat low-fat, high-carb diets often still feel hungry despite a big, hearty high-carb dinner.

Ghrelin, a fast-acting hormone like CCK, is a major appetite-stimulating hormone made by the pancreas and stomach. It triggers immediate hunger, especially cravings for salty and sweet foods that contain unhealthy fats. Levels are lower when you are thin and higher when you are fat. Typically, ghrelin should increase before meals and then decrease after eating. But these levels can get out of whack in response to things like stress, skipped meals (especially breakfast), restrictive dieting, and lack of sleep. Eating—you guessed it—good fats, especially omega-3s, helps to keep ghrelin levels balanced.

All of this is why I have dubbed good fats "sexy, slimming fats."

Now that you understand the "slimming" part of fats, what about the "sexy" part? Outside of how alluring they make your food taste, good fats contribute innumerable benefits to your health, especially to your hormonal health. You need the essential fatty acids from fat in order to *produce* hormones. That's how crucial the sexy, slimming fats are to hormone regulation. You need to make the hormones before you can regulate them!

Fats also facilitate oxygen transportation and assist in the absorption of fat-soluble vitamins A, D, E, and K. Fats make up cell membranes, and cells make up every part of your body. The cell membrane maintains cell structure and controls which substances enter and exit the cell. This has implications for the cell's ability to get rid of waste, take in nutrients, talk to other cells, and receive hormonal messages. Cell membranes need fat to function properly. Furthermore, the brain consists of 60 percent fat. It too requires enough healthy fat to keep in good working order, and to keep your nerves reacting and synapsing. On top of all this, fats really do make you sexier! They fuel sex hormone production and can boost libido.

The point is, when there are not enough fats in your food, you are keeping your body from operating at its best. During perimenopause in particular, you need good fats to help your brain and cells work properly, and in a harmonious hormonal environment.

Types of Fat

Dietary fats have a complex makeup; these include saturated, monounsaturated, polyunsaturated, and even trans fats, with subcategories within each group. Both dietary and body fats are made up of a combination of one, two, or three fatty acids plus a molecule of glycerol, an alcohol. Fats are called monoglycerides, diglycerides, or triglycerides, depending on the number of fatty acids in them. At least two fatty acids—linoleic acid and alpha-linolenic acid—are not made by the body and have to be obtained from food.

The terms "saturated" and "unsaturated" refer to the structure of the fat molecule. Saturated fats have all possible hydrogen atoms present, while unsaturated fats do not. Unsaturated fats are further classified as monounsaturated, when they have one double bond between adjacent carbon atoms, and polyunsaturated, when they have more. A simple way to tell the difference between them is that, at room temperature, saturated fats are solid and unsaturated fats are liquid. Contrary to popular opinion, unsaturated fats do not, as a general rule, have fewer calories than saturated fats, nor are they necessarily better for you. Most fats are a mixture of saturated, monounsaturated, and polyunsaturated, with one kind predominating.

Type of Fat	Room Temperature State	Refrigerated State
Saturated fats	Solid (except tropical oils)	Solid
Monounsaturated fats	Liquid	Semisolid or solid
Polyunsaturated fats	Liquid	Liquid (except when hydrogenated)

Oils are liquid fats, and omega-3, -6, -7, and -9 oils are key suppliers of fatty acids to the body for the manufacture of important hormones. In the next chapter we will look at omega-rich oils (specifically flaxseed oil and black currant seed oil) that provide balm for the female body.

Food Sources of Saturated Fats

Animal Sources

Full-fat dairy products (butter, cream cheese, ice cream, whole milk)

Organ meats

Beef, lamb, and pork fats (suet, tallow, and lard)

Vegetarian Sources

Cocoa butter   Coconut oil   Palm oil

Food Sources of Monounsaturated Fats

Vegetarian Sources

Almonds, almond oil   Macadamia nuts, macadamia nut oil

Apricot kernel oil   Olives, olive oil

Avocados, avocado oil   Peanuts, peanut oil

Food Sources of Omega-3 Polyunsaturated Fats

Animal Sources

Anchovies	Herring	Sardines
Bass	Krill	Shrimp
Cod	Mackerel	Squid
Crappie	Oysters	Trout
Flounder	Sablefish	Tuna
Halibut	Salmon	

Vegetarian Sources

Flaxseeds, flaxseed oil	Nonhydrogenated organic soybean oil
Leafy greens	
Pumpkinseeds, pumpkinseed oil	Walnuts, walnut oil
	Wheat germ
Sea vegetable, fresh	Wheat sprouts

Food Sources of Omega-6 Polyunsaturated Fats

Animal Sources

Lean meats	Mother's milk	Organ meats

Vegetarian Sources

Corn	Sesame seeds, sesame oil
Hemp seeds, hemp seed oil	Nonhydrogenated organic soybean oil
Leafy greens	
Legumes	Spirulina
Nuts and seeds, raw	

Botanicals

Black currant seed oil	Evening primrose oil
Borage oil	

Eicosanoids

The fat in food provides the body with the essential fatty acids necessary to build eicosanoids, hormones that, according to some authorities, control just about every bodily function. They are known to be affected by the nutrients the body absorbs from food. These hormones have lifetimes of less than a few seconds, and prostaglandins are the only type of eicosanoid most nutritionally conscious individuals recognize as a familiar name.

Eicosanoids are assigned to "good" and "bad" categories, although "positive" and "negative" might be better labels since the body, to be healthy, needs both categories in balance. Bad eicosanoids increase on a high-carbohydrate diet, with undesirable results in the body.

Eicosanoid Functions

Good Eicosanoids	Bad Eicosanoids
Blood vessel dilating	Blood vessel constricting
Anti-blood clotting	Pro-blood clotting
Bronchiole dilating	Bronchiole constricting
Immunity strengthening	Immunity weakening
Anti-inflammatory	Pro-inflammatory
Cholesterol reducing	Cholesterol increasing
Pain decreasing	Pain increasing
Antidepressive	____
Endocrine hormone stimulating	____
____	Triglycerides increasing

About 40 percent of calories should be derived from fats for a hormone-regulating diet. Fats supply nine calories per gram.

"Good" and "Bad" Fats

A diet rich in sexy, slimming fats is critical for your health. But which fats are sexy and slimming and which, well, aren't? Some experts say the concern about saturated fat is oversimplified—or even misplaced. Others say we eat too much saturated fat in the United States, and those who eat monounsaturated fat have fewer cardiovascular problems. In truth, whether a fat is good or bad cannot be determined by whether it is unsaturated or saturated. It comes down to the quality of the fat, which depends on its source and its purity.

Let's tackle the biggest myth first, about vegetable oils. So proudly proclaimed as heart healthy on food labels, commercial vegetable oils are in fact low-quality, impure fats, which those labels conveniently omit. First off, vegetable oils are almost always genetically modified, impure from their unnatural laboratory birth. Second, their polyunsaturated structure renders them unstable; they easily go rancid. This means if manufacturers want to use them in many food products, they must process them to avoid rancidity. You will read more about the dangers of processing in a moment, but know that processing fats makes them impure and bad for your health. In addition, because these fats are unstable, they denature in high-heat situations, like the refining process, frying, or other types of cooking, and they oxidize quickly in the body. When a substance oxidizes, it creates free radicals: highly reactive molecules that damage DNA and cell membranes. Cellular damage caused by free radicals has been linked to aging, cancer, and other diseases.

Finally, commercial vegetable oils contain a highly refined omega-6 content. I know—this is a little confusing. Omega fats are supposed to be good for you—and they are. As a matter of fact, omega-6 is an essential fatty acid that is critical to the cell membrane. But when a polyunsaturated fat like omega-6 is refined and non-expeller-pressed, the body cannot use it how nature intended. Instead, the body finds itself unable to utilize the parent linoleic acid of this fabricated fat or to transform it into necessary prostaglandins, like GLA (more about this in the next chapter), and the refined omega-6 fatty acids become inflammatory in the body.

Furthermore, there is a trick to the omega-6: you have to consume it in *balance* with its sister essential fatty acid, omega-3, in order for your body to derive its full health benefits. Ideally, omega-3 and omega-6 fats should be consumed in a 1:4 ratio. In today's food world, with erroneous diet guidelines (I am looking at you, American Heart Association) and the prolific use of vegetable oils in a variety of food products, most people consume omega-3 and omega-6 fats in a ratio of 1:20 to 1:50.

The food industry's addiction to omega-6s has serious repercussions for our health. In 2014, Dr. Rajiv Chowdhury led a team that reviewed seventy-two studies on fat and heart disease, which collectively followed more than six hundred thousand people in eighteen countries. The results fly in the face of the conventional dietary wisdom of the past half century.

The review found that the omega-6 fats in vegetable oils can *cause* heart disease, not prevent it like those "heart healthy" labels claim. According to the report, only one type of omega-6 fat, called arachidonic acid, reduced the risk of heart disease. This type of omega-6 is either produced in the human body or found in poultry, eggs, and beef. The review also showed that omega-3 fats from fish have the most protective qualities of all the fats assessed.

The rest of the review's findings lead me to the second fat myth, about saturated fat. Saturated fat is a neutral fat that will not harm your health and can even provide some benefit. After an incredibly indepth analysis, the reviewers found that butter, a saturated fat, reduces the risk of heart disease, particularly if it is made from the milk of grass-fed animals. Perhaps most importantly, the reviewers also found that two saturated fats circulating in the blood—palmitic and stearic acids—are associated with heart disease. And these fats (wait for it) are manufactured in your liver when you eat carbs.

There is a reason butter is so popular in soul food: it is good for the soul! By "soul" I mean not only the heart but the brain too. Recall that the brain is made of 60 percent fat—and that fat is largely *saturated* fat. Foods rich in brain-building saturated fat include butter, bacon, lard, oysters, liver, and avocados. Some of these foods may strike you as strange. Bacon, butter, and lard have been crucified in the court of public opinion as saturated harbingers of obesity and premature death. But I reiterate: what matters is the quality of the fat.

Animal fats that come from factory-farmed, antibiotic-filled animals are not good for you or your hormones. When you eat fats from these animals, you are consuming the same harmful chemicals they ingested in their cramped, malnourished factory lives. On these factory farms, so notorious for poor living conditions, livestock eat a chemically treated grain diet unnatural to them; depending on the animal, they would typically eat grass, seeds, and small bugs. Animals fed a corn- or soy-based grain diet are higher in omega-6 fats. In addition, factory farmers treat their livestock and the feed with chemicals like antibiotics, growth hormone, and substances that contain dioxin as a by-product, one of the most potent carcinogens known to us. If your steak meal ingested these chemicals, then you will too.

Even if a fat comes from a clean source, such as an organic animal or plant, if it has been processed and/or chemically altered (for example, processed meat and partially or fully hydrogenated oil) it is dangerous for your body. This type of fat is not pure, and its unnatural state leads it to act unnaturally in the body. Furthermore, substances used to alter the fat, like aluminum and nickel, can tag along with their newly bonded fat friend and have toxic effects on the body.

Speaking of altered and damaged fats, partially and fully hydrogenated vegetable fats—which are not the same as trans fat—are also something to be wary of. Food companies hydrogenate fat to keep it from going bad for an unnaturally long amount of time. This saves them money but costs you your health. Bubbling hydrogen gas through a liquid polyunsaturated fat chemically prevents the fat from becoming rancid. However, this hydrogenation process also makes polyunsaturated fat more like saturated fat in molecular structure, and it is no longer in a natural form as food. Plus, as part of the hydrogenation process, a portion of the fat turns into trans fat.

Trans-fatty acids have moved to the black list. They are so dangerous that the U.S. Food and Drug Administration has told food manufacturers to remove them from all products. Trans fats are mostly human-made, naturally occurring only in very small amounts in plant and animal products. Our bodies do not recognize them as nutrients and cannot process them. They clog up the liver and impede its ability to cleanse our bodies of toxins and to burn fat. This hampered detoxification directly leads to hormone imbalances because destabilizing waste products remain in our bodies. This can lead to liver toxicity and, among other things, estrogen dominance since your liver is unable to process excess estrogen and xenoestrogens. (I will include more about estrogen dominance and xenoestrogens in chapters 7 and 13 respectively.)

Consuming trans fats can cause a number of other adverse effects, including

- Lowering "good" HDL cholesterol

- Raising "bad" LDL cholesterol

- Increasing total serum cholesterol levels by 20 to 30 percent

- Lowering the milk volume in lactating females of all species, including humans

- Decreasing testosterone levels in male animals as well as decreasing sperm levels

- Lowering birth weight in humans

- Increasing blood insulin levels in response to glucose load, upping the risk for diabetes

- Altering adipose cell size, cell number, lipid class, and fatty composition

- Escalating the adverse effects of an essential fatty acid deficiency

- Potentiating the formation of free radicals

Don't let food labels trick you. "Trans fat free" means the product contains fully or partially hydrogenated oils, and this should cause your dietary alarms to go off. These foods can contain up to half a gram of trans fat per serving under the regulations of the Food and Drug Administration, and as little as two grams of trans fat can have negative repercussions on your health.

Also beware of oil labels claiming "partially hydrogenated" and "fully hydrogenated." An originally liquid plant fat becomes completely solid when it is fully hydrogenated, essentially turning it into a saturated fat with little trans fat. Partially hydrogenated oils, on the other hand, live in a semisolid middle ground where trans fat abounds more freely. But even if a label says an oil is fully hydrogenated, food companies often mix fully hydrogenated oil with liquid vegetable oil in a process called interesterification. This process makes a new oil product that behaves like a partially hydrogenated oil without the trans fat, yet it still creates a fat that is not pure or natural, and studies have linked it to increased blood glucose and decreased insulin production, which, as you read, can lead to type 2 diabetes. Furthermore, food companies are not required to include "interesterified fat" on the label. Instead, foods that contain fully hydrogenated oil, or high-stearate or stearic-rich fats, may contain interesterified oil.

Now let's talk about canola oil. First off, "canola plants" do not exist in nature. This plant only came into existence through the genetic modification of rapeseed. Unlike other vegetable oils, canola oil has a high level of omega-3s, not omega-6s. However, do not let this omega bait and switch lure you in. Canola oil is a polyunsaturated fat and easily goes rancid, so it must be deodorized to remove any rancid smell before commercial use. The deodorization process transforms most of canola oil's omega-3s into trans fat. Studies have shown that canola oil blocks vitamin E in the body, which protects cells from free radicals and protects the heart. For this reason, you need to cut out the canola.

After reading about all the bad fats, are you ready to meet the good fats? The following is a quick chart of sexy, slimming fats, which I think are especially full of health benefits for not only women during perimenopause but people in general. I will go into more detail about these healing oils in the next chapter, but eating a diet rich in these fats overflowing with therapeutic benefits will promote good hormonal function and overall health. I have also included neutral (neither positive nor negative health consequences) and undesirable (negative health consequences) fats.

Sexy, Slimming Fats

Avocados

Butter (pasture-raised) and ghee

Camelina (wild flax) oil

CLA (conjugated linoleic acid)—from safflower oil and grass-fed whey, butter, and cream

Coconut, coconut oil, and medium-chain triglyceride (MCT) oil

Dark chocolate—in moderation: 1 ounce twice a week

Fatty fish, fish oil

GLA (gamma-linolenic acid)—from black currant seed, borage, and evening primrose oils; hemp seeds and hemp seed oil; and spirulina

Nuts—most varieties, especially almonds, macadamia nuts, and walnuts

Olives, olive oil

Omega-7 (palmitoleic acid)—from anchovies, macadamia nuts, and sea buckthorn

Seeds and seed oils—especially chia, flax, hemp, and pumpkin

Neutral Fats

High-quality saturated fat from grass-fed and organically raised animal protein, such as beef suet, lard, butter, yogurt, milk, cream, and cheese

Undesirable Fats

Fats from factory-farmed, chemical- and grain-fed animals

Processed vegetable oils—canola oil, corn oil, cottonseed oil, and soybean oil

Trans fats

Allison

For about six months, Allison had been losing her hair. At first, the loss had been hardly noticeable—a few extra hairs to be pulled from a comb or brush. Within a couple of months, there were a lot more hairs to be pulled from her comb and brush, plus more caught in the drain after she took a shower. At forty-three, Allison was proud of her shoulder-length jet-black hair, which she wore in a ponytail when active but preferred to wear loose. But now the least bit of pressure pulled it out by the roots. Her husband said it was probably stress from her new job as principal of the local junior high school. Allison felt that, if anything, she encountered less stress in this new position than she had as a classroom teacher.

Then Allison began to notice that the muscles of her thighs and upper arms were becoming less firm than they had been. Her husband asked if her new job was more sedentary than classroom work. It seemed to her that she was never off her feet, rushing from one part of the school to another to resolve an unending stream of minor problems. She was sure it wasn't lack of exercise that was causing her muscles to become flabby.

Her family doctor could find no medical cause for her hair loss or flabby muscles. On the chance that these symptoms might have something to do with an early beginning of menopause, he recommended that she see her gynecologist. Noting that her menstrual cycle was more or less regular, her gynecologist dismissed this possibility. She told Allison to come back the following week when the results of her lab tests would be available. All the results came back normal. At a loss, the gynecologist suggested that she see a nutritionist.

A friend of Allison's had been a client of mine and referred her to me. Determined to find relief, Allison drove more than two hundred miles to see me.

When I asked Allison about her daily diet, I began to see why her gynecologist had recommended a nutritionist. Allison ate what amounted to a vegan diet, with beans and other legumes as her only source of protein. If she had been healthy on such a diet, I would have had little to say. But she was not healthy, not taking the care to ensure she consumed enough plant-based protein and, as I soon found out, did not associate any of her symptoms with her meager diet. In fact, the opposite was true. She was convinced that were it not for her strict veganism, her symptoms would be worse.

Allison didn't have any ethical reasons not to eat animal products. Having heard that vegan women have the strongest bones, she had gone on a vegan diet as an antiaging strategy. I explained that her diet was probably largely responsible for her hair loss and flabby muscles. Allison had a fast metabolism and type B blood, and that could explain why veganism had not worked for her. (Chapter 15 discusses how individual differences influence a person's bodily responses to food.) I suggested that she should eat small amounts of protein at every meal, such as fish, eggs, or organic turkey. As a safety measure, because of her age, I also suggested that she try natural progesterone cream (discussed in chapter 7). In less than two weeks, her hair loss began to ease and her thigh and upper-arm muscles regained some firmness. In six to seven weeks, she was back to normal. Since that time—four years ago—Allison has maintained her health with a protein-rich diet. She remarked to me that she no longer had a tendency to put on weight, although she had never complained of this as a symptom. (Clients so often don't describe all their symptoms!) I said that it was probably due to protein stimulating the hormone glucagon to mobilize body fat to be burned as fuel.

Although physicians increasingly recognize nutrition as a complementary therapy if a patient suggests it, I found it encouraging that Allison's gynecologist had recommended a nutritionist to review her eating habits. Good sign!

Hormone-Friendly Proteins

Hormones and other hormone-like chemical messengers in the body, such as neurotransmitters and prostaglandins, actually are proteins. This is exactly why I call protein "hormone friendly." Proteins are crucial for repairing tissue, improving adrenal fatigue caused by stress, stabilizing blood sugar, and losing weight. Human proteins are made up of twenty-two different kinds of amino acids, nine of which the body cannot make itself and must obtain from food. These nine are thus called essential amino acids. While the body absorbs proteins whole from both animal and plant food, it does not use them whole. Instead, it breaks them down into amino acids and reassembles its own proteins from these. Amino acids are also widely used by the body without being resynthesized as proteins.

The amino acids that make up protein are called the "building blocks of life" because the body uses them to build, rebuild, and repair its tissues and organs. If water were removed from a human body, more than half its dry weight would be protein. Our skin, hair, nails, muscles, hormones, metabolic enzymes, and neurotransmitters are all composed of some of the more than fifty thousand proteins that the body makes use of. Since our bodies don't store amino acids as they do carbohydrates and fat, we need to get a constant supply of these nine

The Nine Essential Amino Acids That Make Up Proteins

Histidine	Lysine	Threonine
Isoleucine	Methionine	Tryptophan
Leucine	Phenylalanine	Valine

essential amino acids in our food. This is another good reason to make sure you get some high-quality protein with every meal.

Proteins perform many life-giving functions inside our bodies. Because of what we have learned about carbohydrates and blood sugar, it's worth pointing out that proteins, like fats, have a stabilizing effect on blood sugar, producing steady, long-term energy instead of a short burst and a quick letdown.

Quite the opposite of carbs, proteins stimulate the secretion by the pancreas of the hormone glucagon, which works in opposition to insulin. What insulin stores in body fat, glucagon puts back into the bloodstream for use as fuel. Glucagon releases the fat-stored sugar glycogen into the bloodstream to restore the blood sugar level and also releases fat from adipose tissue. This fat, burned as fuel, then disappears.

It's interesting to compare the functions of the two hormones:

Functions of Insulin and Glucagon

Insulin	Glucagon
Lowers blood sugar level	Raises blood sugar level
Stores fat	Mobilizes fat from storage
Triggered by carbohydrates	Triggered by proteins

Adult protein requirements tend to be much underestimated in traditional low-fat diets. Approximately 30 percent of calories should be derived from proteins in a hormone-regulating diet. Proteins provide four calories per gram. In the Peri Prescription, you will be satisfied by protein in the form of red meat, poultry, seafood, unfermented and non-GMO soy, whey, beans, eggs, and pea and rice proteins.

Those wanting to lose weight need more protein, especially at breakfast, to help stimulate metabolism throughout the day. Protein builds muscle, and muscle burns fat. When your body has more muscle, it burns fat more effectively, even when you are sitting still.

Do note that restaurants tend to serve double portions of protein, typically around 8 ounces. That size, like most restaurant servings, is simply too big. Learning about portion sizes will help you monitor not only your protein consumption but also your consumption of all the other nutrients when you decide to dine out.

There are many high-quality plant and animal sources of protein, and I have listed a few recommendations in the following list. The most important thing, as I have said, is the quality of these proteins. Just like with fat, protein sources need to be high quality, not filled with chemicals or from factory-farmed sources, and pure, not processed. For this reason, I am adding a caveat to the list: all these protein sources need to be organic, non-GMO, and, for animal sources, pasture-raised, free-range, and grass-fed.

Beans (adzuki, black, garbanzo, etc.)

Beef

Eggs

Fish (wild-caught salmon, etc.)

Greek yogurt

Lamb

Lentils

Pea protein

Poultry

Rice protein

Tofu and tempeh

Whey protein (from A2 non-mutated milk)

A Balanced Diet

Our food needs to be composed of a *balance* of carbohydrates, proteins, and fats. A stable blood sugar level is one of the benefits of a balanced diet. With a stable blood sugar level, a woman experiences fewer health risks and enjoys an even mood, more balanced hormones, extended energy, and greater concentration and attention span.

We've all been hearing about a balanced diet since our schooldays, and I mention it here only because so many of us as adults ignore it. Eating a lot of junk food, as people in the United States do, is putting yourself at risk of an unbalanced diet. Fad diets that deprive your body of nutrients that it requires are certainly unbalanced. Carb-loading for high-performance sports is a deliberate but no less stressful and unhealthful way to unbalance your diet.

For hormonal regulation and sustained physical and mental effort, nothing beats a balanced diet. Your body will let you know when you have reached a dietary equilibrium that works for your specific needs. Your mood will improve, along with your hair, skin, and nails. Your hunger will normalize. You will burn more fat and store less. How great is that?

5.

Getting Personal with the Sexy, Slimming Fats

Boost Metabolism, Brighten Your Mood, and Lower Your Blood Pressure

So now you know that the right kind of fats can help reset your metabolism, stress level, appetite, and sex drive, creating a greater sense of hormonal balance amid the throes of perimenopause. While you have already been introduced to them, on a personal level I want you to become more familiar and comfortable with the sexy, slimming fats—your hormones' new best friend.

The Essentials

Without sufficient quantities of two very special essential fatty acids in particular, your body cannot manufacture all kinds of important substances—including the stress and sex hormones that seem to play a major role in perimenopause. Indeed, essential fatty acids are one of the slick stars of the hormonal health show.

In spite of their name, fatty acids are not themselves fats. They are the building blocks of fats, like amino acids are the building blocks of proteins. They have somewhat similar names, the omega-3 called "alpha-linolenic acid" and the omega-6 called "cis-linoleic acid." In the body, they break down into a series of compounds, most of which have equally confusing names. These fatty acids are considered essential because, unlike the other fatty acids your body needs, the body cannot manufacture these special two. If your very-low-fat diet does not supply enough omega-3 and omega-6 fatty acids for your body's requirements, you are forcing your body to operate at a suboptimal level, especially during perimenopause, while you are already managing the tumult of hormonal change.

The health benefits attributed to polyunsaturated fats are rightfully those of omega fatty acids. Along with the B complex vitamins and vitamin E, the omegas control cell growth as well as help in the manufacture of hormones. Their by-products are ingredients of cell membranes and nerve sheaths. These fatty acids help dissolve body fat, lowering blood levels of cholesterol and triglycerides. They distribute the fat-soluble vitamins A, D, E, and K throughout body tissues. And they are building blocks for prostaglandins.

Perhaps the most important issue to be aware of is that essential fatty acids are not only hormone balancers but also especially anti-inflammatory. Inflammation has been linked to every disease known to us and can destabilize hormones.

Prostaglandins

I mentioned eicosanoids in the previous chapter, the most important of which are prostaglandins. Indeed, the two names are often used interchangeably. You will remember that prostaglandins are very short lived (less than a few seconds), hormone-like substances that control most, if not all, your bodily functions. The better-known endocrine hormones (insulin, progesterone, and so on) are secreted by glands, while prostaglandins seem to be secreted at locations all over the body and by various kinds of tissue.

Among many other functions, prostaglandins are known to stimulate the secretion of hormones, and to alleviate various PMS and perimenopause symptoms.

Prostaglandins can be made only from the two essential fatty acids, omega-3s and omega-6s. From a nutritional point of view, some of the steps from an omega fatty acid to a prostaglandin are useful to know, because the intermediate substances are also available in food.

For example, the omega-3 alpha-linolenic acid (ALA) is found in wheat sprouts, wheat germ, nuts, and seeds—and in their oils. Flaxseeds and walnuts—and their oils—are very rich in omega-3 too. On the path to becoming prostaglandin E3, the parent oil, alpha-linolenic acid, transforms into eicosapentaenoic acid (EPA), a more biologically active form of omega-3. EPA is found in large amounts in cold-water fish oils, from fatty fish such as salmon, sardines, and mackerel, but only in fresh fish, because much of the EPA deteriorates in freezing or canning processes.

As another example, the best sources for omega-6 cis-linoleic acid are unrefined, 100 percent expeller-pressed oils. These oils are produced by pressing seeds, nuts, or vegetables through a screw press at the lowest possible temperatures. Solvents or chemicals are not used, and, unlike refined oils, an unrefined oil is not filtered a second time, deodorized, or bleached.

Cis-linoleic acid can become a prostaglandin in two different ways, either from a second step as gamma-linolenic acid (GLA, another type of omega-6) and then on to prostaglandin E1 or by adding a third step as arachidonic acid (a polyunsaturated type of omega-6) before becoming prostaglandin E2. You can supply your body with ready-made GLA from evening primrose oil, black currant seed oil, spirulina, hemp seeds, and borage oil. Remember, if the oil is refined and non-expeller-pressed, regardless if it is an omega-6 or an omega-3, it becomes inflammatory and is no longer a good source of fat.

Partially hydrogenated vegetable oils and other commercially processed oils and margarine, along with fried food—what I call damaged, altered, human-made fats—can interfere with the transformation of EPA or GLA into prostaglandins. Excess heat, air, light, or hydrogenation in oil processing turns beneficial polyunsaturated fats into harmful substances. On a more general level, a bad diet or lifestyle habits, illness, or medication can interfere with the transition of fatty acids into prostaglandins.

Healing Benefits for Women

So many bodily functions, health benefits, and disorders are associated with the metabolism of essential fatty acids and prostaglandins that an entire book could be devoted to them. We will look at just a few health benefits of special concern to women in their thirties and forties.

- Essential fatty acids, through the prostaglandins they help manufacture, are a prime source of relief from many perimenopausal symptoms by helping to promote effective hormone communication.

- Fish oils containing EPA lower blood cholesterol and triglyceride levels and reduce the stickiness of blood platelets, thereby lowering the risk of blood clots.

- Prostaglandin E3 relaxes blood vessel walls, preventing arterial spasms and lowering blood pressure. Migraine symptoms may be relieved in this way.

- For women who are diabetic or prediabetic, lack of insulin may interfere with the manufacture of EPA or GLA, resulting in a shortage of prostaglandins and symptoms of nerve twitching, infection, and sexual dysfunction. Ingesting oils rich in EPA or GLA may make up for the deficiency.

- Skin, hair, and nails benefit from GLA or EPA in combination with zinc and vitamin A. My clients have noticed an improved complexion, strengthened nails, and a disappearance of dandruff. Eczema, acne, and psoriasis show improvement too.

- Even if you do nothing else in the way of diet and exercise, you can lose up to five pounds by regularly using omega oils in your salad dressings.

- Omega fatty acids combat depression. One analysis of thirteen studies showed the mood-boosting qualities of EPA and DHA (docosahexaenoic acid) to be comparable to that of antidepressants.

- Omega fatty acids also help with hangovers and alcohol withdrawal symptoms—and we all know someone who could use this kind of assistance.

- The essential fatty acids make cell membranes less permeable to the passage of yeast and thus check the spread of infection.

- Fish oils cause tissue changes that may lower the risk of breast cancer. In 2013, a review of twenty-one independent studies found that a diet rich in fish and marine n-3 polyunsaturated fatty acids (such as ALA, EPA, DHA, and DPA [docosapentaenoic acid]) is linked to a 14 percent lower risk of breast cancer.

Food Sources of Omega Fatty Acids

From many studies, it appears that U.S. women do not ingest enough omega-3 fatty acids for their general health needs, let alone enough to alleviate female symptoms. While the majority seem to get enough omega-6 fatty acids, if those are derived from processed or hydrogenated oils, the fatty acids are biochemically impotent. The inescapable conclusion is that women in their thirties and forties need a food plan resembling the Peri Prescription, which is rich in both omega-3 and omega-6 food sources. And if the Peri Prescription is not sufficient to fully treat their symptoms, they need additional omega-rich foods or supplements.

Mother's milk supplies adequate quantities of both omega-3 and omega-6 fatty acids and is one of the few foods to do so, along with flaxseed oil. Cow's milk is a comparatively poor source and skim milk even poorer. To seek additional quantities of the two essential fatty acids in our diet, we need to look at different food sources for each.

Omega-3/EPA Food Sources

Regular meals of cold-water fish and seafood provide enough EPA for ordinary health needs but may not be sufficient to alleviate perimenopausal symptoms. The amounts eaten on the Peri Prescription should be enough to remedy milder symptoms. If your symptoms are stronger,

Percentage of Alpha-Linolenic Acid (ALA) Omega-3, Precursor of EPA, by Total Weight

Flaxseeds, flaxseed oil	58–60%
Perilla oil	54–65%
Black currant seed oil	10–12%
Pumpkinseeds, pumpkinseed oil (Eastern European type)	5%
American black walnuts, walnut oil	5%
Olives, olive oil	1%
Leafy vegetables, fresh (average serving)	0.009%
Chia seed, chia seed oil	0%

Amount of Eicosapentaenoic Acid (EPA) Omega-3 in 3.5-Ounce Serving of Various Fish

Fish	EPA, in milligrams
Anchovy	747
Chinook salmon	633
Herring	606
Mackerel	585
Albacore tuna	337
Pacific halibut	194
Atlantic cod	93
Rainbow trout	84
Haddock	72
Swordfish	30
Red snapper	19
Sole	10

you need to deliberately seek out omega-3 and omega-6 or EPA and GLA food sources and supplements.

Flaxseed oil is the richest source of the omega-3 alpha-linolenic acid (ALA), the precursor of EPA.

North Atlantic sardine oil, at 18 percent EPA, is the richest food source of EPA. This, of course, is not the oil that sardines are canned in but an oil made from the fish themselves. Salmon oil has 9 percent EPA, and mackerel oil has about 5 percent. The fish get their EPA from eating shrimp-like krill, which in turn have eaten cold-water plankton, which use EPA as a kind of antifreeze (plankton in warmer waters are less rich in EPA). In general, the oilier the fish flesh, the more EPA it contains.

Sea vegetables (edible seaweed) and green leafy vegetables are also sources of EPA. Do note that sea vegetables that come from Japan are not a safe option, as the water is contaminated with toxic radiation due to the Fukushima Daiichi nuclear disaster. I recommend getting your sea veggies from Maine or other parts of the northeastern United States. (See Resources for my preferred supplier.)

Fish Oil Capsules

Many of us don't get the opportunity frequently to eat fresh cold-water fish with oily flesh. In addition, fish with high fat contents are most likely to have fat-soluble toxins in their flesh, such as PCBs, dioxins, and heavy metals like mercury and arsenic. Another convenient option to get in your daily fantastic fish fat is to take fish oil liquid or capsules, which tend to come from the oil of anchovies, cod, krill, mackerel, salmon, sardines, or tuna.

Selecting the Best Fish Oil

To be a good consumer, follow a few simple suggestions for finding the highest-quality fish oil capsules.

- MOLECULAR DISTILLATION: Fish oil can be processed by a number of different methods. For the highest quality, look for fish oil that has been processed by molecular distillation. This state-of-the-art process is performed by placing the fish oil on a plate in an evacuated space and heating it. A cold condenser plate is placed as close to the heated plate as possible. Most of the material passes across the space between the two plates, losing very little of its nutritional value but most of the contaminants.

- PHARMACEUTICAL GRADE: There are several grades of fish oil available, ranging from the lowest (cod liver oil) up to the highest (pharmaceutical grade). A typical 1,000 milligram capsule of pharmaceutical-grade fish oil contains at least 600 milligrams of long-chain omega-3 fatty acids. Only pharmaceutical-grade fish oils enable you to consume the required daily intake of long-chain omega-3 fatty acids without fear of environmental pollutant accumulation.

- CERTIFICATE OF ANALYSIS: Environmental toxins find their way into our air and water, where they are incorporated into the fat of small animals, including fish. It is important to minimize your exposure to these potentially toxic substances by selecting a fish oil supplement that has been tested for dioxins, PCBs, and heavy metals. Look for a "certificate of analysis" that confirms the fish oil has passed the tests for environmental toxins.

- TRUTH IN ADVERTISING: A common practice among fish oil manufacturers is to label their product "pure salmon oil" with "18 percent EPA and 12 percent DHA." However, salmon oil contains 6 percent EPA and 9 percent DHA so there is no such thing as salmon oil with higher percentages. To achieve the higher levels, the manufacturer must fortify the salmon with other oils, such as mackerel, sardines, and anchovies.

Please consume only respected brands, as low-quality fish oil can go rancid. In addition, consider performing these three simple tests to ensure the freshness of your choice of fish oil capsules.

1. TASTE: Puncture a capsule with a pin and squeeze a drop of oil onto your tongue. A pure, high-quality fish oil does not taste fishy. A fresh oil tastes mild and sweet. Rancid oil tastes bitter.

2. COLOR AND CLARITY: Light color and clearness indicate freshness and lack of PCB or heavy metal contamination. As fish oil ages, it darkens and becomes cloudy.

3. FREEZABILITY: Put a capsule in the freezer compartment of your refrigerator. If its contents congeal within a few hours, it has a high saturated fat content. The higher the capsule's saturated fat content, the lower its EPA count.

Omega-6/GLA Food Sources

Unrefined vegetable oils are the richest food source of cis-linoleic acid, the precursor of GLA. Other foods rich in this essential fatty acid are green leafy vegetables (such as kale, collard greens, and swiss chard) and brains, kidneys, lean red meat, liver, and sweetbreads.

Percentage of Cis-Linoleic Acid Omega-6, Precursor of GLA, in Various Unrefined Oils

Safflower	78%
Sunflower	69%
Corn	62%
Soy	61%
Walnut	59%
Cottonseed	54%
Sesame	43%
Rice bran	32%
Peanut	31%
Olive	15%
Coconut	2%

Richest Sources of Gamma-Linolenic Acid (GLA), in Various Unrefined, Unaltered Oils

Borage	24%
Black currant	15–19%
Perilla	14%
Gooseberry	10–12%
Evening primrose	2–9%

Omega-7

While omega-3 and omega-6 tend to get all the glory, they are not the only omega fats that have mega health benefits. Omega-7 (palmitoleic acid), although not an essential fatty acid, improves heart health, insulin sensitivity, and cholesterol levels, as well as reduces fatty liver and levels of fat and triglycerides in the blood. It is also one of the most anti-inflammatory omega fatty acids. In fact, omega-7 can cause inflammation markers like C-reactive protein to fall within thirty days by nearly 75 percent. Needless to say, omega-7 fatty acid is a major player in your overall health.

While it's balancing your hormones and healing your health, omega-7 can help you lose that extra perimenopausal weight too. It is the most active fatty acid in regulating lipid (fat) metabolism and has an important say in weight regulation. When observing omega-7 in a petri dish, researchers at Harvard University found that it acts like a fat-burning signal to fat cells—which can become inactivated because of age, stress, or environmental toxins. This omega fatty acid also elevates satiety hormones by over 25 percent, helping you to feel satisfied with less food, thus significantly reducing your caloric intake.

You can find this powerhouse of an omega fatty acid most bioavailable in anchovies and sea buckthorn berry oil, as well as in macadamias and macadamia nut oil. Never heard of sea buckthorn? Allow me the pleasure of introducing you. Much better known by healers in places like China and Europe, sea buckthorn seed oil boasts high levels of antioxidants and the highest levels of natural carotenoids, like beta-carotene, zeaxanthin, lycopene, and lutein. The sea buckthorn berry oil, when used topically, acts as a collagen enhancer to aid mouth ulcers, rosacea, eczema, skin redness, and burns. Sea buckthorn berry oil can also improve gastrointestinal health by reducing inflammation. The two types of sea buckthorn oil are commonly taken together for synergistic effect.

#1 PERI ZAPPER
Flaxseeds and/or Flaxseed Oil

Omega-3s, found in flaxseed oil, are credited with a long list of health benefits, including lowering blood cholesterol levels, helping insulin receptor binding, boosting the immune system, and bettering mineral metabolism. Popular oils, like almond, avocado, olive, peanut, safflower, sesame, and sunflower, while containing varying amounts of omega-6, contain negligible omega-3. Of the readily available vegetarian oils, I prefer two that contain desirable amounts of omega-3 with a healthy balance of omega-6 essential fatty acids. They are as follows:

Oil	Content of Omega-3	Content of Omega-6
Flaxseed	58–60%	18–20%
Perilla	54–64%	14–20%

Quite apart from its qualities as a remedy for perimenopausal symptoms, flaxseed oil also has a reputation as a cancer fighter. It came into prominence through Johanna Budwig's successful use of it with milk as a tumor-reducing medication in Germany in the 1950s. She recommended that 1 or 2 tablespoons of low-fat cottage cheese be ingested with the flaxseed oil to provide sulfur-containing amino acids to interact with it in the body. Its cancer-fighting talent is due to its ability to counteract the destructive effects of refined and processed fatty acids. It's believed that some prostaglandins derived from arachidonic acid (the second of the two omega-6 chemical transitions discussed earlier in this chapter) are cancer promoters. EPA and another omega-3 fatty acid, docosahexaenoic acid (DHA), compete with and displace arachidonic acid in cell membranes. In this way, these omega-3 fatty acids protect the body, particularly against cancers of the breast, colon, throat, and skin.

Author, nutritionist, research pharmacist, and my old friend Ross Pelton claims that the imbalance in our diet between omega-3 and poor-quality omega-6 fatty acids is responsible for many of our growing health problems. He points out that hydrogenation and refining of vegetable oils and processing of grains have caused an 80 percent reduction of bioavailable fatty acids in the U.S. diet over the past hundred years. While Pelton is talking about the incidence of cancer, I have seen a similar effect in perimenopausal symptoms. When women with symptoms restored the balance of healthy omega-3 and omega-6 fatty acids in their bodies, their symptoms evaporated.

Because the Peri Prescription already includes omega-3-rich foods, such as fresh cold-water fish and flaxseed oil, many of my clients on this diet have found that taking an additional tablespoon of flaxseed oil a day is sufficient to get their bodies back in balance. Women not on the Peri Prescription need to take 2 tablespoons a day.

Lignans, the Phytonutrients in Flaxseed Oil

When buying flaxseed oil, look for the kind that is "high lignan." Lignans are a class of phytonutrients that quell perimenopause symptoms as well as quench free radicals and combat the cell-proliferating powers of excess estrogen. Studies continue to reveal the cancer-fighting ability of lignans, especially for hormone-sensitive malignancies like breast cancer. Keep in mind that some breast cancers do not spread, while others grow very slowly. And some tumors are very invasive, spreading quickly to other parts of the body. In some cases, the lignans in flaxseed oil seem able to clamp down on invasive activity. For example, in Toronto, Dr. Lilian Thompson, a leading authority on flax, led a clinical trial involving fifty women with breast cancer. Half of the women were fed flaxseed muffins every day. The women who received this daily dose of lignans had slower-growing tumors compared to the other group.

Another study, completed at the University of Toronto in 2002, compared the effects of flax and soy for their phytoestrogenic properties and ability to protect against breast cancer. Postmenopausal women were randomized into three groups. Two groups supplemented their diet with a muffin containing 25 grams of either flaxseed or soy, and the third group received a muffin with no supplementation.

Urine samples were collected and tested for urinary estrogen excretion. The results are just one more reason why I have said good-bye to soy. The researchers confirmed that flaxseed supplementation exerted a stronger antiestrogenic effect than soy. In fact, flaxseed rivals the power of the anticancer drug tamoxifen, without the adverse side effects.

Indeed, the American Institute for Cancer Research includes flaxseed as one of its "foods that fight cancer," citing multiple studies that prove flaxseed's anticancer properties. In one study, researchers gave flaxseed to postmenopausal women who had just received their breast cancer diagnosis. After only one month of consuming this super seed, the women saw decreased cancer cell growth. Furthermore, healthy women who incorporated flaxseed into their daily diet experienced a decrease in estrogen levels or saw their estrogen converted to a more inactive form.

Consuming lignans helps prevent and treat other hormone-dependent diseases, including heart disease and osteoporosis. In addition to increasing "good" cholesterol and decreasing "bad" cholesterol, lignans protect against bone loss and may increase bone density. Also, studies have shown that people with the lowest rates of several malignant diseases have the highest levels of lignans present in their blood, urine, and feces.

Lignans' secret weapon is phytoestrogens. Phytoestrogens are plant estrogens that experts estimate to be five hundred to one thousand times weaker than human estrogen but can still mimic human estrogen enough to bind with estrogen receptors in the body. By binding with estrogen receptors, lignans help regulate estrogen levels by escorting excess estrogen from the body. This is the reason lignans do so much to prevent and slow down breast cancer as well as improve perimenopause and menopause symptoms. Another interesting quality of lignans is that they have both estrogenic and antiestrogenic activity, meaning they have the power to modulate estrogen to meet the body's changing requirements.

Flaxseeds are nature's most abundant source of lignans, containing up to eight hundred times more plant lignans than wheat bran, buckwheat, millet, oats, rye, or soybeans. Lignans occur in the fibrous shell of the flaxseeds. You can currently buy regular flaxseed oil or high-lignan flaxseed oil in the market.

Finding Quality Flaxseed Products

Please keep in mind that not all flaxseed products are created equal! Buying a quality flaxseed oil from a high-caliber company is one way to ensure that you are getting the best product available. Here are the criteria to use:

- Look for flaxseed that has been grown in the Canadian prairies. These cooler northern climates yield higher levels of alpha-linolenic acid (ALA).

- Remember to check if the oil has been expeller-pressed (also called "cold-pressed"). As I mentioned earlier, expeller pressing is a mechanical process that avoids the use of heat and harsh chemicals. This process results in a higher-quality, more stable oil.

- Another key to high-quality flaxseed oil is organic certification. Organically grown flaxseeds are grown without chemical pesticides, herbicides, or fertilizers. They also have not been irradiated. Be sure to look for a product that has been certified as 100 percent organic.

- Have you heard of vertical integration? This is the system by which flaxseed products can be traced back to the seed from which they were grown. Suppliers who can offer a traceability system show their sincere commitment to producing a quality product.

- GMP (or Good Manufacturing Practices) is another type of certification to look for. These are stringent quality control standards used to provide safe, quality products. GMP processing is important for all EFA (essential fatty acid) oils.

- Beware of genetically modified flax! It does exist. Make sure your flaxseed supplier is willing to verify that its flaxseed is not genetically altered.

- If you buy whole flaxseeds, please remember to grind them prior to eating. This is the only way to release the powerful lignans from inside the seeds. If you consume the seeds whole, they will pass through you undigested.

- It is possible to purchase milled flaxseed, but it should come in a vacuum-sealed package to prevent exposure to oxygen. The package should have a ziplock closure so that you can reseal it between uses.

- Keep in mind that it makes no difference whether you purchase golden or brown flaxseeds. The nutritional content is identical.

2 PERI ZAPPER
Black Currant Seed Oil

The small, round, juicy berries of *Ribes nigrum,* or black currant plant, are familiar ingredients in herbal teas and jams. What is not as well known is that the tiny seeds inside the berries are a rich source of essential fats. Oil produced from black currant seed contains 10 to 12 percent ALA and 15 to 19 percent GLA, gamma-linolenic acid— which is considered the predominant fatty acid. GLA is a precursor for prostaglandins, including the highly beneficial prostaglandin E1, which plays an important role in multiple physiological functions.

Adding a rich source of GLA (like black currant seed oil) to your daily regime is a smart health move. It does, after all, offer relief from those irritating hormone-related symptoms (such as cramps, breast tenderness, water retention, and irritability), gives hormonal production support, and powerfully boosts metabolism.

In addition, the GLA contained in black currant seed oil wears a variety of health-promoting hats:

- IMMUNE BOOSTER: GLA production decreases with viral infection or illness. Supplementing with GLA helps safeguard immune defenses. In fact, when GLA (with EPA) was given to chronic fatigue sufferers, their symptoms improved dramatically.

- CHOLESTEROL REDUCER: A reduction in prostaglandin E1 wreaks havoc on cholesterol levels. Taking 250 to 1,000 milligrams of GLA daily has been shown to increase prostaglandin E1 levels while reducing cholesterol.

- CANCER FIGHTER: In one study, terminally ill patients suffering from pancreatic cancer tripled their life expectancy after taking extensive doses of GLA. It is also believed that tumor growth and metastasis can be quelled with GLA—especially in melanoma and colon or breast cancer.

- ARTHRITIS RELIEVER: Mobility, morning stiffness, and inflammation have all been eased by GLA supplementation, which helps suppress immunity-boosting T-cell proliferation. One study also found that patients were able to reduce their usage of potentially harmful NSAIDs (non-steroidal anti-inflammatory drugs) while they were taking GLA supplementation. Studies have found that effective dosages are in the range of 1.4 to 2.8 grams of GLA per day.

- DIABETIC NEUROPATHY: GLA has been shown in conclusive studies to stop the progression of nerve disease and help with nerve function. Additional studies suggest GLA may even be a catalyst in hindering nerve deterioration at the start.

- METABOLISM IGNITOR: GLA turns on your metabolic fire by stimulating brown fat—adipose tissue that cushions organs and insulates the body—to burn calories, and by stimulating an enzyme-based process called ATPase in which sodium pumps in the cell membranes balance sodium and potassium levels inside and outside the cell. GLA can trigger ATPase to use up to nearly 50 percent of the body's total calories.

- HAPPINESS HELPER: GLA, like other fatty acids, can elevate levels of serotonin, a neurotransmitter that is deficient in a person experiencing depression.

GLA is one of the gatekeepers to not only our health but our aesthetics as well. Beauty-wise, this incredible nutrient really goes all out, flaunting its anti-inflammatory and rejuvenating prowess. It actually increases cell resilience and moistens the fatty layer beneath the skin, delivering a multitude of beautifying benefits, such as

- Producing a dewy complexion

- Aiding against collagen loss

- Soothing dry, scaly skin

- Combating wrinkles

- Nourishing straw-like hair

- Strengthening brittle nails

- Helping to prevent dandruff

GLA . . . it's a health promoter, beautifier, hormone balancer. That triple punch is why black currant seed oil takes center stage as my Peri Zapper #2.

I recommend taking GLA in the ready-made supplemental form because natural sources of parent oils tend to be refined and processed today in food products, blocking their GLA from converting to beneficial prostaglandins and causing adverse health effects. In addition, the average diet tends to lack the vitamins necessary for GLA to convert to prostaglandin, and contains further conversion-blocking agents like trans fat, excessive saturated fat, or alcohol. That's why it is especially imperative to follow the Peri Prescription alongside supplementing with black currant seed oil.

CLA

GLA's cousin, conjugated linoleic acid (CLA) is considered a necessary fatty acid both for cell growth and as a building block for cell membranes. It is also one of the fatty acids that will most help perimenopausal women deal with a slowing metabolism and the resultant weight gain. While GLA targets brown fat, CLA affects visceral fat, the type stored in the abdominal cavity. Excess visceral fat, also called active fat, has particularly dangerous repercussions for hormonal functioning due to its inflammatory nature, and it can increase the risk of glucose intolerance and insulin resistance, which can lead to type 2 diabetes, heart disease, Alzheimer's, and cancer.

In 1997, a ninety-day double-blind clinical study conducted in Norway found that taking CLA with no other dietary changes led to a 20 percent decrease in body fat, with an average fat loss of seven pounds. CLA also increases lean muscle mass and reduces the type of inflammation that causes the breakdown of collagen, which leads to cellulite. You can find CLA in grass-fed dairy foods like butter, cream, and full fat cheese; in beef and lamb; and in capsule form, derived from sunflower oil.

Olive Oil

People around the shores of the Mediterranean have been using olive oil as a nutrient from the times of the Bible and ancient Greece and Rome. Although it has no omega-3 fatty acids and only 8 percent omega-6 fatty acids, this monounsaturated oil is a good source of the most satiating omega fatty acid, omega-9, and the oil has countless health benefits, not all of which are known even after three thousand years of use. Many nutritionists would not be surprised if future research uncovers that olive oil does indeed help alleviate a number of perimenopausal symptoms.

We already know that the oleic acid in olive oil helps prevent the spread of yeast infections. Olive oil also raises levels of the fat-burning hunger hormone adiponectin, is a proven anti-inflammatory, and has been shown to promote neurological, bone, and heart health. And in 2015, in a study conducted at the University of Navarra in Pamplona, Spain, researchers found that women who supplemented their Mediterranean diets with extra-virgin olive oil had a 62 percent lower chance of developing breast cancer when compared to the control diet.

Olive oil comes in three grades: extra-virgin, virgin, and pure. The first two grades are pressed from a single pressing without heat and are therefore desirable. The differences between these two grades lie in the quality of the olives used. Pure olive oil is a combination of refined oils from later pressings and is much inferior. That's why I recommend opting for extra-virgin olive oil when at all possible.

Please be a savvy consumer when purchasing olive oil. Olive oil adulteration is prolific. According to a University of California at Davis study, nearly 70 percent of the fourteen sampled brands of imported olive oil sold in California and labeled as "extra-virgin" failed to meet the extra-virgin sensory standard established by the U.S. Department of Agriculture and the International Olive Council. In reality, the imported Italian extra-virgin olive oil you are purchasing is likely not extra-virgin, nor even from Italy. Too often this olive oil is actually produced in another country (Spain or a North African country) and then shipped to Italy. Once there, some refineries cut it with sunflower oil or soybean oil and beta-carotene, mislabel it, and then send the oil to supermarket shelves across the globe. I have come to trust the California Estate Extra-Virgin Olive Oil, which is the highest in beneficial polyphenols.

Tom Mueller, who wrote *Extra Virginity: The Sublime and Scandalous World of Olive Oil,* maintains an excellent blog that advises consumers on buying quality olive oil.

Snack Fats

Most of the sexy, slimming fats I have described so far, with the exception of olive oil and fish oil, are not as common in daily life and not likely to be on the menu next time you eat out. Have you ever seen black currant seed oil sprinkled on a restaurant's salad? Sadly, me neither. However, there are sexy, slimming fats that are easy to find, quick to prepare, and delicious to eat. I call these the "snack fats" for their on-the-go dose of high-quality fat. Snack fats include coconut, avocados, nuts, and dark chocolate.

From a metabolic perspective, *coconut* can do no wrong. It feeds the thyroid, making it a hormone-regulating superstar, and it is the only source of saturated fat that does not require bile to break it down for your body to use it. Coconut oil actually bypasses the gallbladder. This is great news for anyone with a gallbladder condition or fatty liver.

Coconut is a rich source of medium-chain triglycerides (MCTs), which can improve the efficiency of your thyroid and boost metabolism more than 50 percent. The MCTs in coconut oil are fast burners that create a most efficient food fuel not only for your thyroid but also for your brain, where they can aid cognitive function. In fact, the MCTs produce ketones, substances your body produces when it breaks down fats for energy; these can play a major role in treating Alzheimer's and other neurodegenerative diseases. Coconut oil is also a rich source of lauric and caprylic acids, and acts as an antiviral, antifungal, and antiparasitic, making it a truly clean food.

Do pay special attention to the health benefits of *avocados.* Although not just a snack fat, these nutritional champions pack fiber, protein, and sexy, slimming fat into a single beautifully balanced fruit. They have as much potassium as a banana, are a good source of vitamin E and carotenoids, and have a high chlorophyll content—a natural source of magnesium. Like other omega-rich foods, avocados are anti-inflammatory and can prevent damage to arterial walls, lowering the risk of heart disease and high blood pressure. Their high omega-9 levels make them incredibly satiating. That, along with the boost avocados give to adiponectin, makes them a great weight-loss aid. In addition, avocado oil is by far the best cooking oil, with its robust nutritional content and high smoke point. An avocado a day may very well keep the doctor away.

I'd really be nuts to forget *nuts*. A heaping handful of nuts is a hand full of nutrition. There are a few in particular of these protein-filled, fatty friends that supply an exceptional array of hormone balancing benefits. Walnuts and walnut oil provide a good source of the omega-3 ALA, promote sleep, and reduce the stress hormone cortisol (more about this hormone in chapter 9). Macadamia nuts and macadamia nut oil provide a good source of omega-7, -6, and -3, boost metabolism, increase adiponectin levels, and, with their high oleic acid content, reduce cholesterol and triglyceride levels. Pine nuts contain omega-6 and omega-9, are extraordinarily helpful in healing the entire digestive tract, including the stomach lining, and support the hunger hormones, balancing CCK and increasing adiponectin.

I do have one caveat about nuts. I have found in working with thousands of clients over the years that many individuals have a really hard time digesting them (think gas and heartburn), unless the seeds and nuts are soaked, sprouted, and/or fermented to deactivate enzyme inhibitors. And then there's the issue of aflatoxins (a mold that can be carcinogenic) found in commercially grown peanuts and peanut butter (technically a legume)—as well as other foods.

However, the main concern I have with lots of nuts in the diet is the high arginine content. Arginine is an amino acid that protects the arteries, enabling them to become more pliable, and that's a good thing. On the other hand, too much arginine in the diet—which is easy to achieve when you go overboard with nuts—can feed viral conditions. For this reason, don't get too nutty with nuts. By all means, enjoy them and their numerous health benefits, but enjoy them in moderation.

The same holds true for *dark chocolate*. Dark chocolate has antioxidants; minerals, including magnesium, calcium, and potassium; and healthy fat, including oleic acid. It can reduce bad LDL cholesterol, it lowers the risk for blood clots, and it increases arterial blood flow. But chocolate also has a high copper content and must be consumed in moderation for this reason. I recommend sticking to 1 ounce of unprocessed dark chocolate—at least 60 percent cacao—twice a week.

Now that you have gotten to appreciate your fatty friends, you can see how much they contribute to optimum health—especially regarding your hormones. When your hormones are out of balance, like during perimenopause, you're out of balance. Yet they may be quickly brought back into balance by a lone dietary solution: sexy, slimming fats. Look to the Peri Prescription to discover the scrumptious fats that are so good for your shape.

6.

The Right Peri Vitamins and Minerals

Zapping Anxiety, Insomnia, Bloating, Nervousness, and Irritability

A slice of bread today is far from your grandmother's bread of yesteryear. A century ago, a slice of bread was made from grain that grew in soil rich with a variety of nutrients, free of powerful pesticides and glyphosate-based herbicides. The grain itself had yet to experience genetic modification, and it received little processing before it arrived at someone's breakfast table as whole-grain bread slathered with organic, pasture-raised butter. Today, genetically modified grain seeds with a subsequently increased gluten content grow on factory-like farms in chemically treated soil that has significantly fewer vitamins and minerals. After harvesting, these victims of nutritional burglary are further assaulted as they are processed into refined foods, leaving them bereft of much of their nature-given nutritional benefit.

And it's not just grain. Many fruits and vegetables sprout from genetically modified seeds in similarly depleted soil. If these foods are processed, they can say good-bye to even more of their original nutritional value.

This modern-day nourishment heist has increased corporate productivity and bottom lines but left today's Western diet defective, and deficient in many of the crucial vitamins and minerals the body needs to function properly. For this reason, I sincerely recommend you fortify your diet with vitamin and mineral supplements. While I think you should always try to get your vitamins and minerals from your diet first, it is not always possible with today's dietary landscape. Moreover, the repercussions of not getting these nutrients can be so profound, particularly during perimenopause, that to risk deficiency is not a bet I am willing to take. As you will read, vitamins and minerals influence every aspect of human functioning, from which hormones are released in the body to whether or not your neurons fire or your heart beats.

The vitamins and minerals discussed in this chapter are those that have special significance for perimenopause symptoms. Symptoms such as anxiety, depression, insomnia, fatigue, bloating, and irritability are often the result of low tissue levels of a vitamin or mineral. Two combinations of mineral imbalance are typically the cause of these symptoms: zinc-copper and magnesium-calcium.

The good news about symptoms caused by vitamin or mineral deficiencies is that they can usually be brought under control through simple dietary changes and by taking the proper dietary supplements.

Nicole

Having run twice in the New York City Marathon and once each in the Boston and London marathons, Nicole was a walking—or should I say running?—encyclopedia of sports information: sports injuries, high-performance nutrition recipes, sports superstitions, names of runners who took steroids, herbal infusions for stamina, and much, much more. I listened to her, enthralled and entertained, though sometimes appalled at what athletes believe. Much of her information was good, but some of it was misinterpreted, and sometimes dangerously so. A no-nonsense computer scientist, she was tall and broad shouldered but with a narrow waist and long legs. She moved gracefully and was also athletically fit. She had a keen mind and, like many successful athletes, was a cool observer of her body. At thirty-nine, she was still running about six miles regularly, but no farther because of her work schedule and lack of time for more extensive training.

Now something was wrong, she said. She had been to a physician, who had told her she was developing osteoarthritis. Nicole told the doctor that she suspected it had something to do with her extreme jumpiness.

"Yesterday," she said, "a friend dropped a plate on my kitchen floor and it shattered on the tiles just behind me. I got such a scare from the sound, you'd imagine I'd been in an earthquake. Then I got mad at her. It was only a dollar-store plate, but I felt so furious at her I had to step out into the backyard to avoid cussing her out over that little thing. I managed to control myself yesterday. But I don't always manage, I'm sorry to say." She took a breath and went on, "Now, I told things like that to the doctor and said if I was getting osteoarthritis, it had to have something to do with me leaping a foot in the air when someone drops a pin!"

"What did the doctor say?" I asked.

"She said I was only thirty-eight—as I was then—and so it was too early for my hormones to be causing it. Then she went on about how many athletes, when they feel their bodies aging, have an emotional crisis. I kind of yelled at her, I guess, that I'd never been a professional athlete or even won a big race, and I'd already made adjustments for career and aging without going bananas. Several months passed, and then one day I was running around the reservoir in Central Park on a visit to New York, telling my sad story to this Columbia student I had met a few times previously. She told me what you said about magnesium. So here I am." She gave me a big smile. "I didn't run here. I flew."

I asked if the doctor had administered a serum calcium test. She had. The results had shown that Nicole's blood level of calcium was lower than normal. She had then decided to load up on calcium-rich foods, like broccoli, turnip greens, and bok choy, only to find, on a re-test, that her calcium level still remained low. Her level of 8.2 reminded me of my own levels years ago when I went out of my way to load up on calcium-rich foods (in my case, low-fat cheese and yogurt) and found that my blood level of the mineral had remained low, despite my dietary intake. Hearing of my own experience, Nicole agreed to have a tissue mineral analysis, which showed the exact opposite of her blood test. Her hair sample revealed an excessively high amount of calcium in her tissues, which suggested to me that she did not have a clinical calcium deficiency but was unable to use the excess calcium already present in her tissues (a situation that paralleled my own).

At the same time, she had a low tissue level of magnesium. Based on her report and on the lab recommendations, I suggested that she eat magnesium-rich foods, such as greens, almonds, and beans, and try 500 to 1,000 milligrams of magnesium daily until she took another blood test and tissue mineral analysis in two months' time. That did the trick. Her blood level of calcium had risen from 8.2 to 9.0, and tissue mineral analysis from a hair sample revealed that her tissue level of calcium was now normal, even though she was not taking any calcium supplements and no longer was eating calcium-rich foods.

The high calcium content of the foods she had been eating when she had first come to see me was not being absorbed into her bones because of a lack of magnesium, and the excess calcium in her tissues was affecting her nerves and contributing to her osteoarthritis.

Because, as I said, athletes are such objective reporters on their bodily conditions, I asked her to send me frequent reports on her progress. Her nerves are much better and she seems to be warding off her osteoarthritis. From a newspaper clipping she sent, I saw that she was the first woman across the finish line in a California race the next year.

Magnesium-Calcium Imbalance

Calcium has been demoted—or, at least, calcium supplementation has been. Calcium is one of the least understood nutrients. We are constantly being advised, in the media, to drink milk and eat low-fat yogurt, cheese, and other dairy products, and to take calcium supplements on top of it all to build our bones and avoid osteoporosis. According to the ads and advice, the calcium and vitamin D that these products contain will protect us from becoming frail-boned women who fall and break a hip, and with only an emergency button on a necklace to save us.

It's not quite that simple—largely because the body has a say in all this. The vast majority of U.S. women do not have a true calcium deficiency. But they do have an inability to utilize the excess calcium that is already in their tissues. I know, this may seem confusing, but allow me to explain.

Our bodies are not much different biochemically from those of our Stone Age ancestors. We could live very healthily today on the diet they ate. The only calcium-rich food they had was mother's milk. Animals were domesticated only about ten thousand years ago. Before that, our ancestors managed to get along without dairy products. Why do we need them now? As you may have guessed, we don't—or at least not in the quantities that the ads suggest.

According to a study published in the *Journal of Bone and Mineral Research,* only 600 milligrams of calcium a day will suffice for the average woman. However, the official recommended daily amount of calcium according to the National Institutes of Health for women between the ages of nineteen and fifty is *1,000 milligrams.* That's 400 milligrams of extra calcium. This gross overestimation has dangerous consequences for those who adhere to it, and, unfortunately, it will not increase the amount of calcium the body can effectively use. That's where magnesium comes in.

The bone benefits of calcium do not come from calcium alone but from the interaction between calcium and magnesium and a whole host of nutrient helpers. Your bones and teeth, of course, require calcium, but without magnesium and other minerals, your body cannot properly deposit calcium in hard tissue; as a result, the hard tissue will weaken. Also, excess calcium prevents magnesium from activating thyrocalcitonin, a hormone that directs calcium to the bones, which in turn stops bones from breaking down and aids in bone reformation. Countless studies prove how decisive this magnesium-activated process is. These studies have shown that magnesium, not calcium from the falsely idolized milk, strengthens bones and teeth.

Furthermore, excess calcium is toxic. The gratuitous amount of calcium ingested from supplements and dairy foods can lead to calcification, the process in which excess calcium is deposited in cells, tissues, and organs. It may sound like a relatively benign mechanism, but imagine the hardening meant for your bones affecting your arterial walls. That's exactly what can happen. Instead of strengthening bones, the excess calcium is inappropriately deposited in soft tissue, causing kidney stones, strokes, hardening of the arterial walls (which can raise blood pressure and the risk of heart disease), and stiffening the lining of the bronchial tubes (which can result in asthma). A review of fifteen independent studies indicated that an extra 500 milligrams of calcium per day led to a 30 percent increase in the risk of a heart attack and a 20 percent increase in the likelihood for stroke.

Another good reason for not needing high amounts of dairy products is that the majority of people over age four are lactose intolerant to some extent. Lactose is the sugar in milk, and it is broken down in our intestines by the enzyme lactase. By the age of four, many of us have stopped producing that enzyme. The undigested lactose moves to the colon, where it ferments and causes bloating, gas, cramps, and sometimes diarrhea. The chances that you are lactose intolerant are particularly high if your ancestry is African, Native American, Greek, Arabian, Ashkenazi or Sephardic Jewish, or Asian.

Dairy products contain nine times more calcium than magnesium. That means you need a lot of magnesium from some other source to maintain a proper magnesium-calcium balance if you drink a lot of milk or eat a lot of dairy products. This was no problem for our ancestors, before the arrival of dairy products. They had an abundant supply of magnesium for their modest calcium needs, found in the nuts, seeds, beans, and vegetables they ate. Their bodies had no need to evolve a magnesium-storing mechanism. But because their food was low in calcium, their bodies did evolve to store that mineral. As I said in my book *Your Body Knows Best*, because of this storage mechanism, a little calcium goes a long way in our bodies today.

Please don't misunderstand what I'm saying. I'm not saying that calcium is bad for you or that it doesn't help your bones. I'm saying that in order to have calcium build your bones, you must have enough magnesium to work with it. Magnesium helps calcium absorption and deposition in the bones, where it belongs.

While we enrich our diet with calcium—we even add the mineral to orange juice and ingest a brand of antacids (Tums) for its calcium content—we eat a magnesium-impoverished diet. We eat less magnesium-rich food than our Stone Age ancestors did, such as leafy green vegetables, nuts, seeds, and sea vegetables. Furthermore, the magnesium-rich food that we do eat has less magnesium than it did during most of the course of our evolution because it no longer grows in unadulterated, nutrient-rich soil. With the best intentions, we have created a magnesium-calcium imbalance.

We even add to this imbalance by eating foods rich in sugar and by drinking alcohol, both of which increase magnesium excretion through the kidneys. Almonds have a high magnesium content and would do much to help lay down calcium as bone. But we often don't eat almonds because we think they contain too much fat. It's noteworthy that in looking at populations with diets high in magnesium (Chinese, Indian, and other Asian peoples), neither osteoporosis nor osteoarthritis is as great a health problem as it is in Western cultures.

3   PERI ZAPPER
M 'n' M (Magnesium and Multivitamins)

As I stated in chapter 2, many women's perimenopause symptoms— mood swings, insomnia, anxiety, tissue dryness, and water retention— can be alleviated by a combination of magnesium and multivitamin supplements, including vitamins B, C, and E. Refer to my instructions for this Zapper in chapter 2. When you feel that your hormones are back in better balance, you may be able to cut back somewhat on vitamin C and vitamin E. But read on to hear more about just how vital these vitamins and minerals are to a healthy body.

Magnesium

With all this talk about magnesium, I should probably tell you a little bit more about this super mineral. Think of it as a hormone rescuer. Magnesium has a role in the production and regulation of hormones, preventing excess cortisol, increasing insulin sensitivity, and allowing the production of thyroid hormone. It can help slow aging by reducing oxidative stress, supporting production of the protective antioxidant glutathione, and keeping telomeres (the ends of chromosomes) long, tight, and together, which also reduces the risk of cancer.

Used in emergency rooms to treat heart attacks, this marvelous mineral acts in part as an electrolyte in the body and helps electrical processes like neural communication and the beat of your heart to occur. Your brain and your heart, the most electrical parts of your body, are the two places with the highest levels of magnesium. It is a cofactor in hundreds of bodily reactions and plays a critical role in the utilization of energy, DNA, and vitamin D.

Overall, magnesium helps to relax your body on a cellular level. Called the "original chill pill" by *Psychology Today,* magnesium can improve any malady that involves overstimulated muscles or nerves, such as anxiety, fatigue, asthma, fibromyalgia, and muscle tension. As you can see, you and your cells literally cannot live without magnesium.

A magnesium deficiency can cause perimenopausal symptoms. Because magnesium acts as a sedative within the body, one of the most significant symptoms of a deficiency is a feeling of extreme edginess—which can make sudden sounds send you into a panic. Going easy on dairy products and avoiding foods artificially enriched with calcium should help. Taking a magnesium supplement of approximately 500 to 1,000 milligrams a day will build up your tissue level and help regulate your hormones. And don't forget that magnesium works with vitamin B6 and zinc in very special ways to alleviate a broad spectrum of perimenopause symptoms.

You can easily find dietary magnesium in leafy green vegetables, seeds, and tree nuts, especially spinach, almonds, cashews, peanuts, and black beans. If you feel adventurous, you can also try some "weeds," which are loaded with magnesium, namely nettles and chickweed. Don't feel like foraging on land? Well, the ocean presents a broad mineral-filled frontier. In fact, magnesium is the third most abundant mineral in the ocean. This means kelp and other sea vegetables have high amounts of magnesium that they absorbed from their ocean home. Even a high-quality unrefined sea salt can provide a good source of magnesium.

Some Perimenopausal Symptoms Caused by Magnesium Deficiency

Anxiety	Memory loss
Apathy	Muscle cramps
Body odor increase	Muscle tremors
Concentration problems	Nervousness
Constipation	Perspiration increase
Depression	Urination increase
Irritability	

Just like plants in the ocean, you can get in your daily magnesium by bathing in it. To do this, take an Epsom salt bath. Epsom salt is simply another name for magnesium sulfate, and soaking in it allows magnesium to absorb directly into your skin. Alongside the benefits of magnesium, sulfate in magnesium sulfate helps in the formation of brain tissue and joint protein, and strengthens the digestive tract's walls. Epsom salt baths are also especially helpful for sore muscles.

Michelle

Having heard me interviewed at an online summit, Michelle contacted my office for an appointment. She said she was forty-four and getting married for a second time. As her wedding day neared, she was aware that the occasional bloating she had been suffering from for some years was becoming more frequent. It made her feel uncomfortable. Even her eyelids, she said, were now becoming puffy, and she seemed to be developing breathing difficulties. She was afraid it was becoming a permanent condition. I had spoken about bloating and water retention at the online summit. Could I help her?

When Michelle came to my office a few days later, I saw that she was visibly bloated. She had a warm, sensitive manner and was casually dressed in a T-shirt and faded blue jeans.

When I questioned her intensely about her medical history and lifestyle, as I do all my clients, she told me that a doctor had prescribed pills for her condition a couple of years previously. The pills, whose name she could not recall, had eased the bloating but left her skin dry and scaly, so she had stopped taking them. The pills had probably caused important nutrients to be excreted with her excess fluid, resulting in her dry, scaly skin. The doctor might have recommended that she take supplements with the pills, but Michelle didn't recall this.

She was vague about her eating habits, but she seemed to eat at no fixed times and often mentioned brand-name fast foods. From this, I guessed that she might have a vitamin deficiency, as so many people do with a similar lifestyle. I recommended that she take a multivitamin every day, plus a B-50 complex of activated and methylated B vitamins once a day and an additional 50 milligrams of vitamin B6.

Vitamin B6 proved to be what she needed. After her bloating subsided, I reduced the dosage and had her take the B6 as part of the once-a-day B-50 complex supplement. This was enough to prevent further recurrences. Although I don't believe that she ever completely abandoned junk food, Michelle did make other improvements in her diet, including eating adequate meals on a regular schedule.

But was this perimenopause or simply a vitamin deficiency that could have occurred at any age? In her case, I can't say for sure, but I can tell you what I suspect. I believe that, had she stayed on her vitamin-deficient diet, in due course her B6 deficiency would have been joined by other deficiencies, possibly in magnesium or zinc, and she would have developed other unpleasant symptoms. Women in their late thirties and forties tend to display symptoms from years of unhealthful eating. Such symptoms would be indistinguishable from perimenopause symptoms. We could think instead of perimenopause and a vitamin deficiency as separate risk factors that combined in Michelle's case to produce the symptom of bloating since symptoms result much more often from multiple risk factors than from single causes.

B Complex Vitamins

They may be B vitamins, but they do an A-plus job for your health, especially during perimenopause. B vitamins support general functioning and are necessary for breaking down nutrients as well as utilizing them in the body. They consist of an interrelated group of vitamins, including some familiar food label ingredients: thiamine (B1), riboflavin (B2), niacin (B3), pantothenic acid (B5), pyridoxine (B6), biotin (B7), and folate (B9).

Since the early 1940s we have known that a lack of B vitamins is responsible for a multitude of health problems, especially for women. Without B vitamins, the liver cannot sufficiently perform its hormone balancing act. It needs B vitamins to metabolize hormones, which in turn evens out hormonal levels and prevents estrogen dominance. In fact, Guy Abraham, a pioneer endocrinologist in women's health, found that a woman's liver needs a complete array of B vitamins to change excess estrogen into its metabolically useful form.

Furthermore, a critical biochemical process called methylation requires adequate levels of B vitamins too. This process is vital for the proper function of all the body's systems. It even has the power to turn genes on and off, thereby affecting how your genes are particularly expressed in your body. Plus, it helps repair your DNA on a minute-by-minute basis. Methylation also controls homocysteine (an amino acid that can damage blood vessels), plays an important role in the fight-or-flight response, helps build immunity, supports detoxification, keeps you on an even keel, and tamps down inflammation.

You are more apt to have decreased methylation activity if you have what's called a *MTHFR* (methylenetetrahydrofolate reductase) gene mutation—and I do. This in turn can contribute to histamine intolerance, cognitive issues like ADHD, depression, anxiety, and, most importantly, a hampered ability to detoxify the body. Therefore, keeping the methylation process happy with sufficient B vitamins is crucial.

Vitamin B6

Vitamin B6 (pyridoxine) has often been called "every woman's guardian angel" because of its power to relieve perimenopausal symptoms, particularly water retention and bloating, skin eruptions, mood swings, and even depression and anxiety. High concentrations of B6 increase the synthesis of the neurotransmitter dopamine and inhibit secretion of the milk-stimulating hormone prolactin. This also alleviates irritability and nervous tension. The late Dr. John M. Ellis said that B6 helps prevent and control nausea and toxemia during pregnancy too. Among its other talents, B6 reduces levels of estrogen and elevates levels of progesterone, thereby improving estrogen dominance. Plus, it helps balance tissue levels of magnesium and is important for collagen formation and bone strength later in life, due to its role in amino acid metabolism.

For the normal secretion of serotonin—the brain neurotransmitter that regulates mood, pain, sleep, and appetite—B6 is needed. It has been shown to improve memory, particularly long-term memory, and increases the brain's capacity to store information.

Dr. Leo Galland, a leader in functional medicine, found that most women with yeast infections have problems metabolizing B6 and are therefore deficient in this vitamin. Taking contraceptive pills increases the body's need for B6 and thus can cause a deficiency too. Recently, a lack of this vitamin has been connected to carpal tunnel syndrome as well.

Food sources of B6 include avocados, bananas, fish, green peppers, kale, legumes, liver, meat, nuts, poultry, soybeans, spinach, sunflower seeds, and whole grains.

Michelle's total dosage of 100 milligrams a day was recommended for a limited time for her water retention. Your daily dosage to prevent perimenopause symptoms should range from 50 to 100 milligrams per day, spread out over the day. Your body can best use an activated version of B6 called pyridoxal-5-phosphate, or P-5-P, and while B6 is probably effective on its own, most nutritionists agree that since the B vitamins affect the absorption and metabolism of one another, B6 should be taken with B complex vitamins.

Folate

Dr. Jonathan Wright, founder of the Tahoma Clinic in Tukwila, Washington, and my physician, considers folate—vitamin B9—to be one of the most, if not the most, deficient nutrients, neck and neck with essential fatty acids for the top spot. This vitamin is all about growth and production. It is essential to cell division and the construction and repair of genetic material. Folate supports neurotransmitter generation, including the generation of serotonin and dopamine. It has expansive benefits for cardiovascular health, especially as it relates to the methylation process and its ability to lower homocysteine levels, which are considered hazardous to the heart when elevated.

Sadly, your summer of fun in the sun has a destructive effect on folate in the skin. When sunlight damages skin cell DNA, folate and vitamin B12 rush to the cell's aid to help treat whatever injuries the cell has sustained. This repair process reduces the chance of skin damage, like a sunburn, and the chance that the cell will turn into a cancer cell. However, exposure to sunlight and temperature extremes, including heat, zaps folate from the skin. A lack of folate hinders skin cell repair and, in severe cases, can result in skin cancer. Folate deficiency can also lead to megaloblastic anemia, irritability, fatigue, trouble concentrating, headache, and depression. In addition, folate deficiency in pregnant mothers is notorious for causing birth defects like spina bifida in their developing babies.

Folate is considered preventative of cancer, colorectal cancer in particular. But that is *before* the cancer develops. Do note that once cancer develops, high levels of folate may accelerate its growth. If you have cancer, avoid folate supplementation, but not the many nutritionally robust foods that supply folate, as their nutrients are important to keep your body strong in its fight against this truly terrible disease.

Brewer's yeast is the best source of folate, along with organic liver. Don't know if you can stomach liver? Dark-green leafy vegetables, such as asparagus, broccoli, brussels sprouts, mustard greens, romaine lettuce, and spinach are great sources of folate. You can also try avocado, cantaloupe, green peas, kidney beans, orange, peanuts, and wheat germ. To maximize folate absorption, avoid alcohol because it blocks folate absorption.

When considering folate supplementation, always choose folate, not folic acid. Folic acid is a completely synthetic, oxidized version of natural folate. It is not considered to be equal to folate in nutritional value and is commonly used to fortify food. Unlike its natural predecessor, it may increase the risk of cancer *before* it develops as well as promote cancer growth. Furthermore, those with a mutation in their *MTHFR* gene have a hard time metabolizing folic acid.

Look for methylated folate (5-methyltetrahydrofolate) when picking a supplement. This version of folate is metabolized well in the body, including in the bodies of those with the *MTHFR* mutation, and it carries none of the additional risks of synthetic folic acid. Take at least 1,000 micrograms daily (approximately 1 milligram).

Vitamin E

Itchy skin, a susceptibility to infections, and varicose veins are all symptoms of low levels of vitamin E in your body. For perimenopausal women, vitamin E is a marvelous remedy for vaginal dryness, hot flashes, breast tenderness, and fibrocystic breasts, in dosages ranging from 400 to 1,200 international units per day. Interestingly, many experts feel that, at the cellular level, vitamin E is similar to estrogen and therefore functions as a natural hormone replacement! For women generally, this vitamin promotes heart health, good skin, and overall physical and emotional well-being. Vitamin E suppositories and ointments dramatically soothe vaginal dryness.

The vitamin's natural food sources are high-quality eggs, green leafy vegetables, nuts and nut oils, seeds, and vegetable oils. Diets that eliminate these fatty foods can cause low levels of vitamin E. Evelyn Tribole, Newport Beach nutritionist and coauthor of *Intuitive Eating*, has said that she considers it difficult to meet the RDA for vitamin E while sticking to a low-fat diet. Unless we eat the fatty foods rich in this vitamin, most of us need a supplement.

Iron

Iron is an ingredient of hemoglobin and, in the right biochemical amounts, is a carrier of oxygen throughout the body. It helps to contribute to strong blood and a well-functioning circulatory system, preventing cold hands, fatigue, lusterless hair, and pale skin. When you have iron-deficiency anemia, you feel tired and cold all the time, and have listless hair, pale, dry skin, and dark circles under your eyes. Lethargy, lack of concentration, headaches, and irritability can be symptoms as well. You can become anemic through loss of iron-rich blood in menstruation. Heavy physical exercise, pregnancy, or nursing significantly increases your need for iron. Perhaps four out of every five women who are very active physically ingest inadequate amounts of iron.

Iron deficiency can cause an eating disorder called pica, which involves an abnormal craving to eat substances other than food. David L. Watts, D.C., Ph.D., the founder and CEO of Trace Elements, Inc., once described a woman patient with an eating disorder due to iron deficiency in which she constantly craved paper. Her craving began gradually, without any specific cause that she could remember. Her appetite for paper increased until it became uncontrollable. If she became emotionally moved as she read a book, she ate the pages. She ate the wrappers as well as the candy inside. When she used a tissue, she couldn't use just one—she ate the whole boxful, and then the box. Yet her cure was simple and completely successful: oral iron supplements.

People with pica have craved animal feces, clay, dirt, hair balls, ice, paint, sand, and paper. Its connection to iron is so strong that I have even heard my anemic patients without pica say that sometimes dirt looks appetizing to them.

Iron deficiency can interfere with the proper functioning of your thyroid gland. An amino acid that is converted to the precursor of the thyroid hormone thyroxine is reduced by 50 percent in iron-deficient women. Because of the close relationship of the thyroid gland to the adrenal glands, they may be affected too.

Increased secretion of your parathyroid hormone can also result in iron deficiency. This takes place because the parathyroid hormone increases your body's absorption of calcium, which is antagonistic to the absorption of iron.

While it is desirable for active women who are still menstruating to take an iron supplement, you need to keep in mind that iron is double-edged. Too little can cause anemia, and too much can result in the far more undesirable conditions of heart disease and cancer. In excess, iron is a potent free-radical instigator. Over time, iron overload can result in conditions like arthritis, diabetes, impotence, sterility, premature menopause, cirrhosis, and organ failure. Iron overload can also be caused by a genetic disorder known as hemochromatosis, a condition said to affect one in every three hundred Americans.

We are exposed to iron in a number of unexpected dietary sources. It is added to white flour during the enrichment process and so is contained in most baked goods, like breads, cakes, cereals, cookies, crackers, and pasta. In addition to your hamburger bun, you can find more iron in the burger itself, as it is naturally available in red meat. Iron is also a prominent mineral that is added to many over-the-counter vitamin and mineral preparations. Its absorption is markedly enhanced in the system with vitamin C supplementation.

Women are much more likely to have too much iron after they stop menstruating. The association of too much iron with heart disease brings up an interesting possibility. Because women's rate of heart disease starts to equal that of men after menopause, estrogen has been thought to be the protective factor in preventing heart disease in women before menopause. This may not be true. The real protective factor may be the monthly loss of iron-rich blood.

Obviously, if you no longer menstruate regularly, you should not take iron supplements. I suggest that as soon as you stop menstruating, start monitoring your ferritin level, which measures the iron stored in your body. You do this through a blood test on visits to your doctor. In this way, you can assess whether iron buildup is a problem you need to be concerned about. If tests indicate that you have iron buildup, you will need to avoid iron-rich foods and multivitamins to which iron has been added.

The best food sources for iron are beans, beets, dark-green leafy vegetables, eggs, liver, and red meat. For perimenopause symptoms, you need 15 milligrams of iron a day if you are menstruating regularly. Pregnant women need twice that. You'll find that taking vitamin C dramatically increases your body's absorption of iron. Red wine and dark beer also increase iron absorption. On the other hand, antacids, aspirin, caffeine, and some food preservatives interfere with iron absorption.

Recommended Daily Values of Some Important Vitamins and Minerals During Perimenopause*

Vitamin B6	2 mg
Vitamin B12	6 µg
Vitamin E	30 IU
Calcium	1,000 mg
Iron	18 mg
Magnesium	400 mg
Zinc	15 mg

*Remember that the FDA's Daily Values were established to prevent deficiency and do not necessarily represent the amounts needed for optimal health.

#4   PERI ZAPPER
Zinc

Remember that zinc helps to balance estrogen and increase progesterone levels. It also builds strong bones, keeps your immune system strong, and fights off viruses—a must for vegetarians, whose diet is often lacking in this vital mineral.

It should be noted that, even though I have been putting copper through the wringer, when in a bioavailable form, copper greatly improves your functioning. It supports vital enzymes in the body and can cause some metabolic mayhem when deficient. Would you believe me if I told you, after all I have just said, that you may have both too much copper *and too little*? Well, bear with me. Many people do have too much *unbound* copper, creating the zinc-copper imbalance and copper toxicity I have described. This copper is not bioavailable for the body to use. On the other hand, many people also have too little *bound* copper. Important copper-dependent enzymes use this bioavailable kind of copper to catalyze reactions and keep the body working. Adrenal stress caused by excess calcium, iron, phytates, vitamin C, and high-fructose corn syrup as well as environmental stress results in this duality of too little and too much copper. Following the general supplementation rules I have outlined in this chapter and the Peri Prescription should restore both bound and unbound copper to their optimal levels.

Zinc-Copper Imbalance

Zinc is of particular importance to perimenopausal women for bone formation. This mineral assists in the absorption of vitamin D and is essential for osteoblast (responsible for bone formation) and osteoclast (responsible for bone reabsorption) formation. Research studies on women of various ages have shown that zinc supplements help slow bone loss as well as boost compromised immune systems. Zinc supplements have recently been shown to fend off certain viruses too, including the common cold. If you have low tissue levels of zinc, you are more likely to have perimenopause symptoms.

Tissue mineral analysis from hair has revealed that women with low zinc levels are likely to have high copper levels. In general, women in perimenopause tend to be copper heavy and zinc deficient. Zinc is closely associated with progesterone, which decreases during perimenopause. When the level of zinc rises or falls, so does progesterone.

Likewise, copper levels seem to rise or fall in tandem with estrogen levels. So we can say that perimenopausal women tend to be both progesterone and zinc deficient. These women usually have too much copper in their tissues and tend to be estrogen dominant. If their progesterone levels were adequate, their progesterone would counteract the effects of the estrogen and they would not have symptoms. Raising your zinc level with supplements and lowering your copper level through dietary vigilance could be the practical solution you are looking for.

Possible Symptoms from Low Zinc/ High Copper Ratio

Constipation	Heavy menstrual flow
Depression	Menstrual irregularities
Fatigue	Mood swings
Food cravings	Weight gain
Frontal headache	Yeast infections

The interesting thing is that low zinc/high copper symptoms are shared by perimenopause and copper toxicity. You can blame either one without ever being sure which is actually responsible, or whether they are jointly responsible. Controlling the nutritional imbalance may be enough to cure the symptoms. But all too often I have to convince clients that symptoms like menstrual irregularities, which they associate exclusively with female hormones, can have both a nutritional source and a nutritional cure.

In discussing zinc-to-copper ratios and similar matters, we need to keep in mind how the human metabolism varies from person to person. What upsets one woman goes unnoticed by another. Needless to say, the fact that one woman doesn't experience any symptoms doesn't make those symptoms any less real for the woman who does. In addition to personal differences in metabolism, other factors in our individual lifestyles can make us more prone to certain symptoms. For example, vegetarians in general are more likely to have copper overload and consequent perimenopause symptoms.

What causes a zinc deficiency to develop? First and foremost, stress. The next most common cause is a diet rich in sugar and processed carbohydrates. After that come vegetarian diets, which omit meat and eggs, both good sources of zinc. Medications are a common cause too. For instance, antidepressants, diuretics, and anti-inflammatory medications such as cortisone and prednisone suppress your body's absorption of zinc, speed its excretion, or interfere with synergistic nutrients, such as vitamin B6 and magnesium. Alcohol is another cause of zinc deficiency, because it increases the excretion of the mineral through the kidneys. Grains, especially those in unleavened bread, have high levels of phytates. The phytic acid in such food binds with zinc and makes it impossible for your body to absorb it. The high fiber in vegetarian diets also causes zinc deficiency.

Too much zinc in your body, on the other hand, causes "bad" cholesterol (LDL) levels to rise and "good" cholesterol (HDL) levels to drop.

Tissue mineral analysis of hair samples is an excellent measure of zinc content in your body over time. However, neither tissue mineral analysis of hair nor the more traditional blood tests can reliably spot an acute zinc deficiency right now. The only reliable way to detect an acute deficiency, in my opinion, is through a person's positive response to zinc supplements.

To get more zinc, enjoy plenty of protein-packed foods, like beans, eggs, grass-fed beef, kelp, lamb, mushrooms, oysters, poultry, pumpkin-seeds, raw cheese, seafood, sunflower seeds, and yogurt or kefir. Vegetarians should definitely consider taking zinc supplements! If you have perimenopause symptoms, you need zinc supplements amounting to 15 to 50 milligrams per day.

Where does the copper come from? According to the late chiropractic physician and researcher Dr. Paul C. Eck, diminished activity of the adrenal glands is probably the most important physiological cause of high copper levels. Adrenal gland activity is required to stimulate production of ceruloplasmin, the leading copper-binding protein. With diminished adrenal activity, the liver makes less ceruloplasmin and unbound copper starts to gather in various tissues and organs. Tissue mineral analysis shows that 70 to 80 percent of women have weak adrenal glands. Other sources of copper include the following:

- The mineral occurs naturally in drinking water in some parts of the country and may be added as copper sulfate to municipal drinking water and swimming pools to eradicate fungi, including yeast.

- Vitamin and mineral supplements often contain copper at levels harmful to some women.

- Vegetarian diets, high-soy diets, corn oil, margarine, mushrooms, organ meats, shellfish, wheat germ and bran, and yeast are all rich in copper.

- Copper water pipes and cookware are sources present in most U.S. homes.

- Birth control pills and copper intrauterine devices supply copper to the body, as do dental fillings, crowns, and other dental appliances.

- People who work with metal, such as plumbers and welders, are at risk of absorbing toxic levels of copper.

Some Foods with a High Copper Content, in Milligrams per 100 Grams

Oysters	17.14
Lamb liver	5.60
Yeast, dried	4.98
Tea, bag	4.80
Cocoa powder	3.57
Soybeans	1.17
Curry powder	1.07

Women cooking with copper-lined pots and pans, drinking water out of copper pipes, or using copper IUDs or birth control pills are at higher risk for copper toxicity. Foods like black teas, chocolate, nuts (especially cashews), seeds (especially sunflower), shellfish, and soy are naturally copper rich.

If you feel that you are over-consuming copper in foods, it is important for you to find supplements that are copper-free. With this caveat in mind, I formulated a copper-free, hypoallergenic multiple vitamin, mineral, glandular, and herbal product called Female Multiple for Uni Key Health Systems (see Resources).

Vitamin D

No conversation about hormonal balance, especially during perimenopause, is complete without vitamin D, which itself is actually a steroid hormone. This potent mood booster, nicknamed the "happy vitamin," has few dietary sources and mainly comes from sunshine. It is produced by the interaction between direct ultraviolet rays and your skin. Vitamin D is fat-soluble, so if you find vitamin D in your diet, it will typically be found in fatty foods. Sources include beef liver, cheese, egg yolks, fatty fish and fish oil, and even mushrooms, which seem to be the only nonfat food source rich in vitamin D.

The steroid hormone D has a close relationship with two other steroid hormones important to perimenopause: testosterone and estrogen. It increases testosterone production, which in turn can lead to increased libido, red blood cell production, and muscle mass, as well as weight loss. A study at Johns Hopkins University published in 2009 found that low levels of estrogen intensify the effects of long-term vitamin D deficiency, increasing the risk of heart disease and osteoporosis.

Like magnesium, vitamin D supports calcium absorption, helping to create strong bones. Vitamin D is so integral to bone health that vitamin D deficiency can lead to osteoporosis, osteomalacia, and rickets, all of which involve weakened bones. It also plays a role in cell growth, neuromuscular function, and the immune system, and can lower inflammation. Emerging results from animal and epidemiological studies suggest that vitamin D can prevent and improve metabolic conditions, such as both types of diabetes and glucose intolerance, as well as other conditions like hypertension and multiple sclerosis.

As it stands, the RDA for vitamin D is 600 international units per day. However, in 2014, research from the University of Alberta showed that the official RDA of vitamin D from the National Academy of Medicine is significantly lower than needed to maintain a healthy body. According to the researcher's statistical analysis, the RDA should actually sit at 8,895 international units per day to ensure that the vast majority of the population has adequate vitamin D in their system. The researchers do note that this dose is higher than any previously studied dose and caution should be taken when interpreting this number. Nevertheless, the bottom line is that the current RDA for vitamin D is much too low. I recommend a daily vitamin D intake of 2,000 to 5,000 international units.

It was previously thought that vitamin D supplementation was necessary in diseases commonly associated with vitamin D deficiency, like autoimmune disorders. A study conducted by researchers from the Autoimmunity Research Foundation, the U.S. Public Health Service, and Cornell University shows that is not the case. The deficiency is actually caused by an infection with the bacteria that live in the body. These infected bacteria in turn make the vitamin D receptors malfunction, impairing the immune system and making people more vulnerable to additional infections as well as encouraging the progression of their disease. Supplementing with vitamin D only exacerbates the receptor malfunction instead of fixing the deficiency. If you have lupus, rheumatoid arthritis, sarcoidosis, psoriasis, type 1 or type 2 diabetes mellitus, scleroderma, Sjögren's syndrome, autoimmune thyroid disease, ankylosing spondylitis, Reiter's syndrome, or uveitis, please limit your vitamin D intake, as any excess of vitamin D can hinder your treatment.

Tissue Mineral Analysis

Nicole's case history in this chapter shows the importance of using tissue mineral analysis of a hair sample to assess mineral levels in tissues that differ from those found in the blood. A hair sample reveals what has been going on in the body for three months, whereas blood constantly readapts to more immediate and short-term metabolic shifts. While I fully acknowledge that many practitioners dismiss hair analysis, I have consistently found it the missing link in subclinical assessment of mineral levels.

Hair analysis provides an accurate reflection of the body's mineral needs when you consider the following: Hairs develop in skin follicles. As the hair cells grow in the follicle, they are exposed to blood, lymph, and extracellular fluids. Once the hair emerges from the follicle, its outer layers harden and thus lock in place the metabolic products that are present. This provides a lasting biological record of the metabolites that were present when the hair emerged.

To find out how to order a tissue mineral analysis, please refer to the Resources section.

7.

Natural Hormone Cream

Fighting Fatigue, Listless Libido, Irregular Periods, and Osteoporosis

Many of my clients find that the Peri Prescription and Peri Zappers #1 through #4 (Flaxseeds and/or Flaxseed Oil, Black Currant Seed Oil, Magnesium and Multivitamins, and Zinc) clear up their perimenopausal symptoms quite simply, but they are not enough for everyone. It's true that the Peri Prescription helps stabilize your body's hormonal balance, and Peri Zappers #1 through #4 should make up for missing nutrients, but everybody is different and has different needs. If the Peri Prescription and these Zapper nutrients don't prove powerful enough to alleviate your symptoms, my next recommendation is to use natural progesterone as a skin cream.

Progesterone is a hormone involved in female sexual behavior, pregnancy, and menstruation that is produced in the ovaries, the placenta, and the adrenal glands. Known as the "feel good hormone," progesterone is up to twenty times more concentrated in the brain than in the bloodstream. This hormone functions as a stabilizing force, counterbalancing estrogen. It has numerous positive benefits, including promoting fat burn, helping to normalize blood sugar and cell oxygen levels, and acting as an antidepressant.

As menstruation slows during perimenopause, so does the production of progesterone. The decline in progesterone means the body now lacks some of its estrogen-equalizing force. This imbalance contributes to some of the nastier symptoms of perimenopause, such as decreased libido, depressed mood, and hypothyroidism-like symptoms such as fatigue and weight gain.

The truth is, these days having a progesterone deficiency seems to be common among all women aged eighteen to eighty. Many women lack the necessary nutrient precursors for their body to produce progesterone, especially zinc and vitamin B6. This only exacerbates the consequences of dropping progesterone levels during the change before the change.

The Menstrual Cycle

To highlight the role of progesterone, let's review some familiar information about the menstrual cycle. A cycle normally lasts twenty-six to twenty-eight days. The cycle begins with the brain sending a message to the ovaries to stimulate egg follicles. Only one egg fully ripens and moves, in its follicle, to the outer surface of the ovary. On ovulation, the follicle bursts, and the released egg travels down the fallopian tube to the uterus.

As the egg is ripening in the ovary, the lining of the uterus walls thickens and develops a network of blood veins. This is in expectation that the fertilized egg will become implanted on the lining and require nourishment. Only a fertilized egg becomes implanted. In the absence of a fertilized egg, the uterine lining is shed and menstruation begins. The cycle then begins again.

For a week or so after a woman's period, estrogen is the dominant hormone. It stimulates the buildup of the uterine lining.

On approximately the twelfth day after a period begins, estrogen levels peak and begin to drop, just before a woman ovulates. After ovulation, the empty follicle that held the egg starts to produce progesterone. The follicle is now called the corpus luteum ("yellow body"), and its progesterone is the dominant hormone of the second half of the menstrual cycle. Progesterone also stimulates the buildup of the uterine lining.

If the egg is not fertilized, both estrogen and progesterone levels drop sharply. If the egg is fertilized, the progesterone level remains high.

If ovulation is missed in a menstrual cycle, there is no empty follicle to become the corpus luteum. Therefore, progesterone is not secreted by the ovary in sufficient quantities to counteract the effects of estrogen, and a hormonal imbalance—and consequent symptoms—result. This condition is referred to as estrogen dominance, alluding to the specific hormonal imbalance that occurs as a result of low progesterone. The term was coined by the late Dr. John R. Lee, whose pioneering work has helped us understand the varying effects of estrogen and progesterone as well as the characteristics of estrogen dominance.

In his landmark book *Natural Progesterone,* Dr. John R. Lee shared an intriguing story about the ancient Celts and their use of mistletoe in their celebration of the winter solstice. In the dead of European winter, when the land was otherwise bleak, non-deciduous oaks persisted in the production of their waxy, white mistletoe berries. During the winter celebrations, the Celts painstakingly harvested these berries from the oaks using white cloths to make sure the plant-born pearls never touched the ground. The Celts then combined the mistletoe berries with hot mead (an alcoholic beverage) to make a sacred intoxicant in which they indulged for the celebration. The celebration was known for its lively intermingling of the sexes, which the aphrodisiac brew no doubt invigorated.

The European mistletoe berry has a high concentration of progesterone. Folk healers took advantage of this progesterone, using mistletoe as a "morning after" therapy for pregnancy prevention. It is also why the mistletoe enjoyed in the Celtic celebrations without a doubt stimulated libido. And because an abrupt fall in progesterone level leads to menstrual shedding, the decrease in excess progesterone the women experienced when they stopped drinking the mead prompted menstrual bleeding, so their sexual engagement likely produced few pregnancies.

Perhaps you now can appreciate not only a potential explanation for why we still today kiss beneath the mistletoe but also the power and potential of some five thousand plants that contain substances similar to progesterone.

Comparison of the Effects of Estrogen and Progesterone

Estrogen	Progesterone
Stimulates uterine lining cell growth	Stabilizes uterine lining cell growth
Stimulates breast cell growth	Stabilizes breast cell growth
Adds to body fat	Helps burn body fat as fuel
Promotes water retention	Diuretic
Promotes depression	Antidepressant
Causes headaches	Does not cause headaches
Anti-thyroid hormone	Pro-thyroid hormone
Promotes blood clotting	Stabilizes blood clotting
Diminishes sex drive	Increases sex drive
Upsets blood sugar balance	Stabilizes blood sugar balance
Anti-zinc and pro-copper in body	Stabilizes zinc-copper balance in body
Lowers cell oxygen levels	Normalizes cell oxygen levels
Raises risk of uterine cancer	Prevents uterine cancer
Raises risk of breast cancer	Helps prevent breast cancer
Anti-bone building	Pro-bone building
Antivascular	Provascular

Characteristics of Estrogen Dominance

Bloating	Mood swings
Breast swelling	Periods—irregular
Depression	Periods—occasionally heavy
Fat deposition on hips and thighs	Sex drive diminishment
	Sugar cravings
Hypothyroid symptoms	Tiredness

Uterine fibroids   Weakened bones

Water retention   Weight gain

The Highs and Lows of Progesterone

Besides its ability to counteract the undesirable effects of estrogen, progesterone functions as both buffer to and treatment for various ailments. It has been credited with fighting heart disease and cancer. For women in their thirties and forties, progesterone plays an active role in bone density; a high progesterone level is a major protective factor against later osteoporosis.

By increasing body energy, probably by helping thyroid hormones work better, progesterone causes a very slight but often noticeable rise in body temperature during ovulation, contributing to enhanced metabolism. This varies from woman to woman.

Because progesterone plays a promotional role in so many functions critical to a good quality of life, such as mood and libido, normal fluctuations in this hormone can have potentially deleterious effects. After a fertilized egg settles on the uterus wall, ovarian progesterone cares for it. After the placenta develops, it, too, secretes progesterone. Progesterone levels continue to be high throughout pregnancy, which is why many women in the third trimester, and in spite of some physical discomfort, feel as good as they have ever felt in their lives. Unfortunately, when progesterone levels fall sharply after the birth, the mother is vulnerable to experiencing postpartum depression.

At menopause, the drop in progesterone level is twelve times greater than that in estrogen level (estrogen declines by 40 to 60 percent). Men have higher progesterone levels than some postmenopausal women. Just like women after they give birth, this drop in progesterone can create a feeling of depression for both perimenopausal and menopausal women.

If you have hair loss and skipped periods, a low progesterone level may be the culprit. Lack of ovulation in a skipped period can cause the adrenal cortex to secrete the hormone androstenedione as an alternative chemical precursor for the manufacture of other hormones to compensate for the diminished level of progesterone. This steroid hormone is associated with some male characteristics, one of which is male-pattern baldness. When you raise your progesterone level with natural progesterone cream, your androstenedione level will gradually decline and your hair will grow back normally. Be patient—hair growth is slow and it may take several months before you notice a difference.

There are also a number of other beauty and health issues that can originate from low progesterone. On a superficial level, the consequences of low progesterone include growing whiskers on the chin, thinning hair, breaking capillaries, gaining weight, and emerging skin problems, such as acne, liver or age spots, and dryness. Internally, it can cause yeast infections, irritability, irregular periods, and mood fluctuations.

Natural Hormone Cream

Luckily, because a fluctuation in progesterone level at least in part causes some of the uncomfortable symptoms of perimenopause, it can also be used to fix or prevent that fluctuation and other maladies.

As Dr. Lee wisely noted more than two decades ago in *Natural Progesterone,* "Age is not the cause of osteoporosis; poor nutrition, lack of exercise, and progesterone deficiency are the major factors." For a woman, osteoporosis typically starts in her mid-thirties, about the time her progesterone level begins to drop, and then accelerates for three to five years after she reaches menopause. The use of natural progesterone—along with a healthful diet, proper supplementation, and exercise—has been shown to be beneficial in increasing bone mass in these women, giving them strong bones into their eighties.

Natural progesterone therapy may relieve a number of issues affecting women in perimenopause. Vaginal dryness and atrophic mucosa (shrinking mucous membranes) are not only unpleasant but also increase the likelihood that women will develop vaginal, urethral, and urinary bladder infections. Risk of infections like pelvic inflammatory disease also increases when vaginal mucus is somehow impaired. Natural progesterone may ease or eliminate vaginal dryness and atrophic mucosa after three or four months.

Ovarian cysts arise when ovulation cannot occur or reach completion. The cysts may disappear on their own or they may progress to the point that they require surgery for removal and possibly the sacrifice of the ovary. As you know, progesterone is crucial to the menstrual cycle. For this reason, the use of natural progesterone from day ten to day twenty-six of the menstrual cycle inhibits stimulation of an ovarian cyst. After just one or two monthly cycles using progesterone, the cyst will likely disappear without any other more invasive medical assistance. Women have experienced similar resolutions of mild to moderate endometriosis, which can be extremely painful and can otherwise require treatment as drastic as a hysterectomy. In the case of endometriosis, women generally must continue the application of natural progesterone for three to five years, or until menopause.

Fibroid tumors, which are not cancerous, are an upshot of estrogen dominance. They can cause heavy bleeding, painful bleeding, and, over time, a dropped uterus and trouble controlling urination. By helping to reverse estrogen dominance, the use of natural progesterone often prevents the tumors from growing, keeping them at bay until after menopause, when they begin to atrophy on their own.

Camilla

Camilla, forty-four, came to my office asking for an energy-boosting diet. She complained of a total lack of energy, chronic tiredness, and constant fatigue. Her doctor had suspected hypothyroidism, but the results of her T3 and T4 blood tests indicated that her thyroid gland was functioning normally.

Camilla understandably thought that maybe the kind of carbohydrate-loading regimen that powers professional athletes would give her more zest. I warned her that every blood sugar high on that kind of diet was followed by an even bigger low.

During our consultation, I soon found out that because of family tragedies, Camilla had undergone a high amount of stress in the past few years. In an almost accidental aside, she mentioned that she used estrogen patches. She hadn't filled that in on the form at the doctor's office as medication she was taking because she had gotten the patches from a friend and didn't consider them medication.

As I saw it, she had become fatigued due to extended stress. Someone gave her the patches as a tonic. The estrogen interfered with the action of her thyroid hormones at the cell receptors, and she developed hypothyroid symptoms, which she may have been predisposed to anyway. I got her to throw out the patches and apply natural progesterone cream to her skin to rebuild her reserves. In three weeks, her major symptoms were gone. She still wasn't ready to run a mile, but now she had some energy. I suggested that she reduce the cream to minimal use, and with the Peri Prescription, supplements, and exercise, she soon became her take-charge self once again.

Natural Progesterone vs. Synthetic Progestin

As a natural substance, progesterone cannot be patented, trademarked, or otherwise protected in the marketplace. It belongs to everyone. In order to make commercial progesterone into a prescription item, pharmaceutical companies deliberately alter the natural structure of the progesterone molecule and come up with a synthetic product called progestin. This strategy may work well in the marketplace, but it does not work as well in your body. The altered progestin you are prescribed functions much less effectively than natural progesterone in your body.

The synthetically altered progestin molecule resembles progesterone enough to mimic the hormone, binding to the same cell receptor sites as the actual hormone and relaying messages into the cell. However, this message is never quite the same as that of natural progesterone, and your body does not process it the same way. You may lose your temper more often, feel increasingly irritable and, at times, emotionally unstable. Progestin can intensify all your symptoms. Because progestin does not match your body's chemistry exactly, it can inhibit ovulation or suppress your body's own secretion of natural progesterone.

Integrative and functional medicine physicians have found that a combination of natural or bioidentical progesterone and estrogen more effectively minimizes symptoms than a combination of synthetic progesterone or progestin and estrogen.

One would only have to look at the *Physicians' Desk Reference* to see the possible side effects of Provera (medroxyprogesterone acetate), the most common progestin. It lists abnormal uterine bleeding, breast tenderness, galactorrhea (milky nipple discharge), hives, itching, edema, rash, menstrual changes, change in weight, mental depression, insomnia, somnolence, dizziness, headache, and nausea. Women taking progestin with daily oral conjugated estrogen may experience an increased risk of developing dementia, ovarian cancer, and invasive breast cancer.

Your body also has difficulty in breaking down progestin and excreting it. This creates a potential for toxic effects, such as heart conditions from unexcreted, partially broken down waste circulating in the system.

Christina

Sometimes a low level of progesterone can have more far-reaching consequences than just feeling off within your body. It can affect the quality of your relationships as well.

"I was a wild girl in Catholic school. I hated the rules," Christina told me. "We had to wear a school uniform. When we got out of school, I always hiked mine up so it was a miniskirt. I can't remember a time back then when I wasn't boy crazy." She sighed at the memory and added defeatedly, "But that was then."

Christina, a stockbroker, had a magnetic personality deftly highlighted by her expressive face, with a pert nose, blue eyes, wavy golden hair, and generous smile. At forty-three, she was gregarious and instantly likable, but her state of mind was not as sunny as her manner led people to believe.

"My husband and I are having some problems," she said. "He's having a lot of late evenings at work. I know that everyone has to work harder just to keep up nowadays, but I know that's not why he stays out. I think he prefers facing a computer screen to facing our relationship."

Christina said the spark was gone—but only her spark. Her husband still lusted for her as he did in college, but Christina now had a hard time reciprocating. As we talked, I couldn't help noticing that Christina felt more comfortable talking about her lack of sex drive from her husband's point of view than from her own. I mentioned this to her.

She nodded. "I've been listening to his complaints long enough. I don't know how to answer. I don't know why, but now I just don't feel it anymore. No matter how much I want to."

Christina had been to a doctor, where she'd had a blood test of her hormone levels. Her estrogen level had come back normal, as had some other levels whose names she couldn't recall (probably FSH and LH). From her test result, the doctor had assured her that she didn't have a hormone problem. Nor did she have any sign of a medical disorder. The doctor had concluded that her loss of interest in sex was probably due to an emotional or psychological problem.

"I know my body, and this didn't feel psychological," Christina said confidently. "I have friends who have struggled with the same thing for psychological reasons, and I feel different from them. The thought of sex doesn't repulse me. I just don't care. I'm indifferent. Not me really— my body is indifferent."

Christina was a bit surprised, I think, when I dropped the subject of sex and started asking her about apparently unrelated symptoms. No, she didn't have weight gain. She wasn't particularly irritable or nervous. In fact, just the opposite. She felt sluggish, especially in the mornings. No headaches. Food cravings? Don't even mention the words. In the last couple of years she had become a coffee and pastry addict. She found that they helped her get going in the morning. A large café latte and a blueberry or cherry sweet roll helped her through her afternoon sinking spell. And she often had coffee and apple pie with women friends when her husband had to "work" late.

I asked if her periods were regular.

"For the past three years or so I've had several very light ones in a row, followed by a heavy one, and then more light ones," she said. "But I've never missed a period."

It was clear that this information seemed unimportant to her. Yet all the pieces of the puzzle were there; she, like so many others, just didn't see how they connected. But her instincts were good, as they are in many women. She had instinctively felt that in her case her body was more a cause of her troubles than her mind. I told her that in this she was almost certainly correct.

Although Christina didn't have some of the more typical symptoms of estrogen dominance, such as weight gain (particularly around the abdomen, hips, and thighs), water retention, irritability, and depression, she had one of the most important classic signs: decreased sex drive. This was probably caused by her not ovulating and consequently lacking corpus luteum secretion of progesterone. The resulting estrogen dominance was responsible for her loss of sex drive, or libido.

After telling her that she first would have to break her caffeine habit and sweet tooth, I put her on the Peri Prescription. In addition, I recommended natural progesterone cream for her to rub on her skin in order to build up and stabilize her tissue level of progesterone. The higher level of progesterone would counteract the libido-diminishing effects of estrogen.

Christina spent some months falling off the caffeine and sugar wagon, and she couldn't really stay on the Peri Prescription until she had broken those habits. During those months, however, she faithfully used the natural progesterone cream on her skin as recommended. Gradually, she began to feel a bit more frisky in the bedroom. Last I heard, she was on the diet and feeling like the girl who used to hike up her uniform skirt in high school again. And her marriage improved too. Finally able to reconnect with her husband, he didn't put in all those evening hours at work anymore.

Natural Progesterone Cream

The word "natural" when applied to progesterone doesn't mean exactly what it sounds like. Here, the term "natural" means that the plant progesterone molecule used to make the cream is identical to the human progesterone molecule, distinguishing it from the pharmaceutical progestin, whose molecule is slightly different from human progesterone. Some creams use extracts from soybeans (which are also used for phytoestrogens); others are based on the wild yam (*Dioscorea*).

You need to be selective when buying a cream, because some creams contain only a tiny percentage of progesterone or none at all. Although a number of creams make claims for it, research has shown that the natural plant form of diosgenin, the active ingredient in yams, does not bind with human cell progesterone receptors, meaning that these creams are useless as progesterone sources.

Diosgenin has to be processed in a lab into progesterone. Some of the creams that contain diosgenin from wild yams also contain lab-grade progesterone, and some do not. Investigators have shown that creams containing only wild yam extract do not significantly boost a woman's progesterone level. On the other hand, they have also shown that creams that contain lab-grade progesterone do boost the body's progesterone level.

#5 PERI ZAPPER
Natural Progesterone Cream

Progesterone cream balances estrogen dominance symptoms, such as decreased sex drive, depression, abnormal blood sugar levels, fatigue, fuzzy thinking, irritability, thyroid dysfunction, water retention, bone loss, fat gain, and low adrenal function.

Picking the Cream of the Crop

Test your hormone levels to learn where your hormones may be out of balance before you start any natural hormone supplementation. Some healthcare professionals will recommend a saliva test. A salivary hormone test, done at home, evaluates your body's levels of bioavailable progesterone, estradiol, estriol, testosterone, DHEA, and cortisol.

In a normal menstrual cycle your body produces 20 to 24 milligrams of progesterone a day for twelve to fourteen days. This comes to a total of approximately 250 milligrams of progesterone for each menstrual cycle. A 2-ounce tube or jar of 1.6 percent (by weight) or 3 percent (by volume) cream contains about 950 milligrams of progesterone. Half of such a tube or jar, applied externally, should provide more than enough progesterone for one menstrual cycle. Apply a total ⅛ to ¼ teaspoon to start, in one or two applications daily. After a week or more, apply a total of up to ½ teaspoon cream daily if your symptoms require it. You may apply the cream as often as you like, so long as you don't exceed the daily total. Also, to avoid saturating the subdermal receptors beneath your skin in any one area, creating dermal fatigue, apply the cream to different areas each day.

When applying, massage the cream into the soft, capillary-rich skin of your face, neck, upper chest, breasts, inner arms, palms and backs of hands, and soles. The progesterone from skin cream is absorbed transdermally into the fatty layer beneath your skin. You will probably notice your skin becoming more resilient and moist in the areas where you often apply the cream. The progesterone is taken from the fatty layer beneath your skin by the bloodstream, which distributes it throughout your system. This is not an overnight effect. It may even take several weeks, or occasionally a couple of months, for the progesterone level to build in tissues and make its effects felt. But don't try to rush the process by taking bigger doses. Too much of any hormone at one time can have the opposite of the desired effect. As progesterone accumulates, it may disrupt other hormones.

The natural progesterone cream that I originally created for myself and then shared with my personal clients is called ProgestaKey (see Uni Key Health Systems in Resources). Many other suitable creams are readily available in health food stores or online. The two that I am most familiar with besides ProgestaKey are Pro-Gest and ProgesterAll.

Even though I think a cream is by far the best delivery method, natural progesterone also can be taken orally, vaginally, or injected. When progesterone is taken orally, most of it goes through the liver, which eliminates up to 80 percent of the usable hormone from the body by either breaking it down or expelling it. Some progesterone oral supplements are in micronized form, which ensures that they will not be largely lost when processed by the liver, and will have fewer side effects concerning the liver. Lozenges dissolve in the mouth, allowing the body to absorb progesterone through the mucous membranes. This can cause a sharp increase in progesterone followed by an equally sharp drop. This dramatic change does not necessarily lead to optimal hormonal balance.

In a world with so many toxic environmental assaults on your body, simply changing your diet alone is not always enough. As you now know, supplementing your well-being with vital things like progesterone can make the difference between a body out of whack and a body on track.

8.

Making All the Right Moves

Discover the Routine Best Suited for Your Body

When your blood sugar becomes stable on the Peri Prescription, your blood level of the hormone glucagon becomes elevated. Whereas insulin adds to body fat, glucagon helps burn it away as fuel for energy. The great thing about having a high glucagon level is that it means you are burning body fat even when you are not physically active—even while you sit here reading this page, even while you sleep in bed!

Obviously, you burn off much more body fat if you are active. You use up more body fat as fuel, measured in calories, as your metabolic rate increases. This has been known for many years, and most traditional diets are based on this concept alone. The new generation of diets that take the body's hormones into consideration has completely transformed dieting, making it progressive and informed. Nutrients evoke hormonal responses from the body, and the hormones then control how the nutrients are put to use in the body.

It's now recognized widely that exercise also evokes hormonal responses from the body. Aerobic exercise reduces your insulin level and elevates your glucagon level. Anaerobic exercise, such as strength training, causes the body to secrete human growth hormone. This hormone, a builder and repairer of muscle tissue in adults, is the great white shark of fat burners. Glucagon promotes vasodilation, the expansion of blood vessels, so that more nutrient- and oxygen-bearing blood can reach muscle tissues and bear away lactic acid when leaving. But fat-burning hormones are not the only ones that respond to exercise. In fact, exercise is one of the healthiest, most effective, and most natural ways to combat depression or stress. This is because exercise releases endorphins, neurotransmitters that heighten mood (which I'll discuss more in the next chapter).

For many years I have noticed how exercise helps just about every symptom of perimenopause. This undoubtedly is related to exercise's hormone-regulating benefits. It reduces cortisol, promotes the production of neurotransmitters like dopamine, serotonin, and endorphins, and promotes the production of testosterone. All of this lowers stress, regulates emotions, and reduces cravings for carbohydrates, as well as boosts metabolism, circulation, and energy level. In addition, exercise is one of your most valuable tools to manage blood sugar and increase insulin sensitivity.

In my experience as a nutritionist, I have noticed that exercise also enables your metabolism to work better and more intensely, so you benefit more from whatever nutrients your body is processing. Although I cannot pinpoint a certain biological mechanism to explain this phenomenon, healing oils, vitamins, and minerals all seem to be more intensely absorbed by the body when you exercise regularly. This means that symptoms are alleviated or disappear faster.

When your body is reasonably fit, most of your bodily systems are in fairly good balance. When only your hormones are out of balance, and the rest of your body is more or less in balance, the Zapper nutrients are free to work on your hormone problem. But if your bodily systems are sluggish and you are out of condition due to a sedentary life, those Zapper nutrients will probably be utilized somewhere else in your system before they ever reach your hormones!

Take It Low and Slow

Now, you've heard me sing the praises of exercise for alleviating perimenopause symptoms, but these benefits apply only to *light* to *moderate* exercise. Overly strenuous exercise, on the other hand, can actually damage the body, increasing stress and all of stress's dangerous consequences. Overexercising—meaning continuous strenuous exercise for two or more hours—can throw estrogen levels out of whack and lead to bone loss, especially during perimenopause. It increases oxidative stress, which, in turn, creates free radicals that can lead to premature aging, heart attacks, cataracts, infections, and a number of cancers.

Nowadays people are being encouraged to do five minutes of gardening, fifteen minutes of walking to the store, pushing a stroller, playing with a dog, raking leaves. It all adds up. You burn a similar number of calories walking briskly that you do jogging.

Much of the really worrisome overexercising that I have seen involves young girls being encouraged by their parents to excel at sports. What makes it heartbreaking is that the young girls usually do it out of fear of disappointing their overzealous parents. But some women in their thirties and forties also suffer from too much physical activity, far more often than you might imagine. However, their activity is rarely sports related. When I think about overexertion, Cheryl comes to mind.

Cheryl

Cheryl, at thirty-eight, had two teenage kids and a husband who had trouble holding down a job. She herself worked full-time at her job of nine years, and in addition she drove the kids to practices and appointments, helped them with schoolwork, cooked, cleaned, did yard work, and regularly checked on her husband's widowed mother, who had diabetes and lived alone. Her husband spent a lot of time away from the house, "looking for work," and usually got home for dinner, flopping into an easy chair. Cheryl felt constantly fatigued and thought I should put her on a special diet.

"What you need," I offered, "may not be a nutritionist but more moderation in your life. Perhaps your husband could pitch in more."

She immediately started defending her husband, saying what a special kind of person he was and how hard he found it to adapt and so forth. While she was talking, she got out of her chair and started tidying up my office. I was preparing for a speaking engagement, and I had arranged papers on the floor. Cheryl picked them all up, placed them neatly on shelves, and sat down again, all the while talking to me. I looked at her and realized that she was not conscious of what she had just done.

Even before discussing her other symptoms or testing her for clinical deficiencies, it was obvious to me that her overriding problem was one of overdoing. She was an overachiever, trying to be a superwoman. With no help from her husband, she was overextending herself. I told her so, and she walked out of my office. I never saw her again.

Housework is exercise. Housework often is intense exercise. Taking care of young children is always exercise. You'd be surprised how many women worry about not having energy enough to go jogging after a day packed with more physical activity than most professional athletes have.

#6 PERI ZAPPER
The Right Moves

Moderate exercise has been shown to help all our bodily systems, including those systems affected by perimenopause. To help maintain health and quell perimenopause symptoms, be moderately active for a half hour five days a week. Do housework, garden, walk briskly, do yoga, cycle, swim, dance, take a Zumba class, have fun. Do different things each day to help keep your mind and body always adapting and flexible, and to prevent boredom. Overall, just do what gets you moving and makes you smile.

Sitting: As Bad as Smoking?

Back in the day, our ancestors had to worry about dying at the hands of a predator. Today, we have to worry about dying at the legs of a chair. Like smoking during the mid-1950s, few people realize how bad prolonged periods of inactivity are for their health. For this reason, an abundance of health experts and news articles have proclaimed sitting to be the new smoking. And I have to agree.

As a matter of fact, in 1991, a British Heart Foundation report implied that lack of exercise was a health risk equivalent to smoking a pack of cigarettes a day. The fact that sitting is an insidious killer is not new information. Nevertheless, researchers continue to look into the impact of the current sedentary living revolution. Over and over again they find that your likelihood of dying from any cause increases with the number of hours you spend sitting on a daily basis.

Our bodies are intrinsically made to move. When we deprive them of that movement, we experience a near universal encumbrance on our bodily systems. Without the stimulating movement of muscles, circulation slows down. This causes fluid to accumulate in the legs, leading to swelling, varicose veins, and blood clots. Likewise, the brain does not receive the full supply of blood and oxygen it needs, creating brain fog. As a result, the brain cannot as effectively carry out its function as one of the main hormone regulators, which spells bad news, especially for women in menopause and perimenopause. Bodily stagnation causes cells to have greater insulin resistance, which has been theorized to promote cell growth and lead to an increased risk for breast, endometrial, and colon cancer. Even the basic position of sitting damages the body in excess. Your muscles wilt as your hip mobility is reduced, your abdominal muscles atrophy, and your glutes weaken. The lack of movement causes your body to burn less fat, which leads to a higher chance of high blood pressure, high cholesterol, and heart disease. The fat accumulation in the blood and its associated risks are only further compounded by the poor circulation caused by prolonged sitting.

With so many of us working eight-plus hours a day at a computer, and then spending an hour or more each night on the couch, it is imperative that we find a way to work extra steps, stretches, and physical activity into our daily routines. If you can, stand for at least two minutes every hour. Leave your desk and walk around for five to ten minutes every hour or so. Stretch your hip flexors every day by resting one knee on the floor and extending the other foot out in front so that your thigh and calf are in an L shape. Even simple cow and cat yoga poses will improve your back's flexibility.

If you work at a desk all day, invest in a good ergonomic chair that supports your lumbar spine and head so you avoid curling your body forward, which strains your neck and accelerates forward-head syndrome. Sit up straight. Keep your feet flat on the floor, the keyboard near your lap so your elbows bend at ninety degrees or wider and your wrists do not arch or strain.

Better yet, invest in a height-adjustable desk that allows you to switch between sitting and standing as you work. Desks such as those made by Varidesk allow you to change their height so you can switch between sitting and standing. I recommend you split your day fifty-fifty, spending half the day sitting and half the day standing. This allows you to maintain your productivity while still mitigating the effects of prolonged sitting.

If there is anyone who understands what too much time spent in a chair can do to the body, Kimberly does.

Kimberly

A sedentary occupation and a fixation with soft drinks are dual problems for U.S. women of all ages. It takes a lot of lifestyle changes to beat that combination. But every bit of exercise helps create that change, so I told Kimberly.

It did no good. So far as I could estimate, Kimberly drank three to four liters of Coca-Cola a day. At her job as a telemarketer, where she often put in twelve-hour days, she ate anything that happened to be around, such as pizza slices, candy bars, doughnuts, or even someone's salad if they didn't want it. She apparently never actually purchased food. And of course she never exercised. At forty-one, she lived at her own apartment sometimes, and at other times, she stayed with her seventysomething mother or with her boyfriend, both of whom lived near her. The only things that weren't vague in Kimberly's life, so far as I could see, were her perimenopausal symptoms.

Her migraines were totally debilitating, sometimes lasting for days, during which she would lie in bed in a darkened room, trying various over-the-counter remedies in what sounded to me like dangerous amounts. They didn't provide her lasting relief, but she tried them over and over again. Insomnia, fatigue, and occasional crawling skin sensations rounded out the picture. Nothing that I recommended seemed to help either—if, that is, she really followed my advice, which I never knew.

Then Kimberly got downsized, in both senses of the word. Out of her present job and interviewing for another, she became frustrated and wanted to create a positive change in her life. She came to see me now on a weekly basis, and I was amazed each week to see the improvement in her. Having lost about fifteen pounds in two months, she had started cooking for herself and buying new clothes. I figured that she was walking about two hours a day, and drinking one liter of Coke.

"Don't go back to telemarketing," I pleaded.

"I thought I might get a job as a bookkeeper or secretary," Kimberly said.

I shook my head. There had to be something else, something active, and there was. She now delivers and installs office telephone and computer network systems. On her feet all day, she must be fifty pounds lighter than a couple of years ago. She follows the Peri Prescription and takes M 'n' M supplements. Except for an occasional headache that passes within a few hours, her perimenopause symptoms have disappeared. Before she started getting exercise, neither diet nor supplements had brought her any relief. I suspect this was because her blood sugar was so unstable—she may have been on the verge of type 2 diabetes—that her system was not metabolizing nutrients very well. Exercise got her metabolism, and her life, going again.

Vigorous Walking

Moderate exercise has been shown to help all our bodily systems. Walking a mile a day has been found to reduce women's risk of losing bone density as they get older. A minimum of four hours of exercise a week reduces the risk of getting breast cancer by 37 percent, researchers found in a study of twenty-five thousand Norwegian women.

Brisk, vigorous walking is the most convenient form of exercise for most of us. For walking to qualify as beneficial exercise, it must be vigorous, so make sure to move your arms. In hot weather, you can walk early in the morning or after sundown. In cold weather, bundle up, or get on a treadmill. If you walk vigorously for thirty minutes or so five days a week, I guarantee you will feel better and look better in a matter of a few weeks.

Walking your way to feeling and looking better is simple. You don't need special equipment, just a comfortable pair of shoes. You can walk alone or with friends. You can vary your route so you don't get bored. As you walk, you can pray, meditate, or plot. You can listen to music (no cellular phone, please, except as an emergency or safety measure).

So if walking is so easy, what's stopping us? Why don't more women walk? Because we haven't got time. Ask anyone. There's really only one answer to that objection. You have to make time. You do that by examining the structure of your days, finding that half hour somewhere, and then treating it as seriously as you do your other duties and appointments. Apart from personal and family responsibilities and your job, how many other activities of your day are as important as getting rid of perimenopause symptoms? Exercise will really help you do that if you give it a chance.

High-Intensity Interval Training

For the many women who live by tight schedules and are in search of a quick, vigorous exercise, high-intensity interval training (HIIT) can pack a big cardiovascular punch into a short amount of time. HIIT consists of alternating intervals of all-out exertion and little to no exertion. Studies have shown a short period of HIIT to be as equally, if not more, effective as thirty to forty-five minutes of moderate exercise in increasing cardiovascular and respiratory fitness as well as providing many of the other benefits of exercise, like increased metabolism and insulin sensitivity.

There are a lot of ways to practice HIIT. You can play with the interval duration and number. I have seen people succeed using intervals of thirty seconds to one minute, alternating between all-out exertion and light movement for a total of ten to fifteen minutes.

Pamper Your Pelvic Floor

The pelvic floor is exactly what it sounds like. It is quite literally a floor of muscle that spreads across the bottom of your pelvic bones, stretching like a trampoline from the pubic bone to the tailbone and from side to side. Strong pelvic floor muscles support your bladder, bowel, and uterus, and help stabilize the hip joints. Supporting the pelvic floor muscles is especially important in perimenopause to give you that reassuring control you want over your bladder and bowels. As an added benefit, a strong pelvic floor improves sexual performance!

Kegel exercises can help strengthen the pelvic floor. To identify the right muscles, stop urinating midstream. You just used your pelvic floor muscles! To do Kegels, the Mayo Clinic suggests you contract your pelvic floor, keep it contracted for five seconds, then release and relax the muscles for five seconds. Do this for four or five repetitions. Over time, build up to ten-second periods of pelvic floor contraction, followed by a ten-second period of relaxation.

Another excellent practice is the deep squat. It will help you keep your pelvis properly aligned. To do a deep squat, simply start squatting, and don't stop until you have gone as low as you possibly can, with your thighs completely on your calves if this is comfortable for you. This is a primal sitting position that you often see young children do. To really get the full pelvic strengthening benefit, pee in this position when you are in the shower. You will activate your pelvic floor in the most natural way possible, the way it was typically activated for thousands of years before indoor plumbing. This positive peeing causes your pelvic floor to stretch and tone.

If you are a little squeamish about going in your shower, practice a deep squat with heel support. Roll one end of a yoga mat up and place it beneath your heels, placing the balls of your feet slightly wider than hip-distance apart on the unrolled other portion of the mat for stability. Focus on using your glutes rather than your quads to deeply engage the pelvic floor. The straighter you can align your shins over your feet, the better. Then lower your bottom toward the mat, place your palms together in front of you, and press your elbows inside your knees. You may have to practice to get into a deep squat. The longer you stay there, the more it will help your muscles and release any tension.

Bounce for Bone Health

Remember jumping on a trampoline as a kid? Little did you know, you were doing wonders for your health. Now a type of exercise called rebounding combines the joys of the trampoline with the joys of good health. This jumping exercise moves and stretches every cell in your body, supporting the influx of nutrients and the elimination of waste as it boosts blood circulation and lymphatic drainage. It also strengthens bones gently without the jarring impact on the joints that more strenuous exercises, like jogging, can inflict.

In fact, in the early 1980s, NASA conducted research that showed rebounding provides a more even, full-body workout than running, with less impact on the body, while still producing similar cardiovascular results.

Exercises to Prevent Osteoporosis

Do keep in mind that some kind of resistance or weight-bearing exercise is needed to prevent osteoporosis. When muscles experience resistance, it creates torque—a twisting force—in the muscles equal to the force it is resisting. This torque then sets off a small but critical electrical impulse that triggers calcium deposition, therefore strengthening in the long run the exact bones being taxed in the moment. To create this necessary resistance for your body, try walking, running, bicycling, aerobics, light weight lifting, or any other form of exercise that makes extensive use of the legs and hips. Twenty minutes to an hour three times a week is adequate. Research has shown that women who did this kind of exercise for an hour three times a week increased their bone density by 2.6 percent in one year.

In particular, strong lower back muscles have been associated with increased spinal bone mineral density in women aged fifty-eight to seventy-five. In other words, a strong lower back means strong spinal bones. To make sure these muscles stay in fighting form, practice good posture and implement back exercises in your resistance training routine.

The Mayo Clinic conducted a study on a type of a safe, progressive resistive weight-lifting exercise that produces impressive results in the lower back muscles. In the study, postmenopausal women ranging from fifty-eight to seventy-five years old lay on their stomachs wearing weighted backpacks equivalent to 30 percent of the maximum they could lift. They then lifted the backpack by lifting their arms, chest, and chin off the floor a total of ten times. They did this exercise five days a week over the course of two years. The amount of weight they lifted increased as their strength grew, with the total weight of the backpack never exceeding fifty pounds. The women who completed the exercise regimen not only strengthened their back muscles during the study but also had less muscle loss eight years later compared to the control group. In addition, their ten-year risk of spine fracture was reduced by 300 percent in comparison to the control group.

An especially effective form of whole-body osteoporosis-preventing exercise is called whole-body vibrational training. Supported with research conducted by NASA, whole-body vibrational training uses 3G Vibration platforms that vibrate at a specific speed to take advantage of gravity. This vibrational motion triggers muscles to use natural reflexes to respond much like if you were unexpectedly falling and trying to catch yourself. Essentially, this stimulates the strong muscle contraction of bracing against a fall—without actually falling. Simply standing or holding different positions on these platforms sends vibrations throughout the body, which stresses the muscles and generates muscle- and calcium-building torque, but without the risk of falling inherent in traditional exercise.

Remarkably, one study showed that using vibrational training actually reversed bone loss, increasing hip bone density by 1.5 percent. Weight training, on the other hand, failed to reverse bone loss at all, making vibrational training more effective at preventing osteoporosis than time spent lifting weights at a gym. In addition, multiple studies have shown whole-body vibrational training to be as effective as weight training in improving muscle strength and balance.

As for me, well, I hate to admit it, but I've never been an exercise enthusiast. I much prefer working to working out. To get my needed sweat session in, I've found success doing a style of exercise called SuperSlow. It uses a very precise method that delivers noticeable results with short workout times and nominal risk of injury. This method was created in the 1980s by a man named Ken Hutchins while conducting osteoporosis research at the University of Florida.

It uses—as you'd imagine—extremely slow movement, focusing on proper form. A sample exercise would be a biceps curl, performed by slowly curling up for ten seconds and then slowly curling down for ten seconds. This reduced acceleration and momentum improves muscular loading because it limits the amount of force your body is exposed to during exercise—unlike more traditional methods. Emerging research shows it to have comparable results to other exercise programs when done consistently for at least ten weeks. Plus, the one to two sessions per week schedule is something even those who typically dread exercise can stick with long term.

The bottom line is, no matter what exercise program you decide to follow, the key is to . . . keep moving!

9.

Taking the Distress Out of Stress

Finding a Place of Calm— Even on the Busiest Days

Overweight, exhausted, sick, and moody? It may sound like perimenopause I am describing, but I am actually talking about stress. Few things are more destabilizing to your health than excessive stress—and it is epidemic in modern society. It lies at the heart of almost all physical, mental, and emotional ailments, and disrupts hormonal function.

As a matter of fact, you could consider stress the body's hormonal reaction to a threatening circumstance. The stress reaction uses a flurry of hormones—crucially, cortisol—to ready your body to quickly utilize its resources and fight or flee the stressful situation. In conjunction with perimenopause, the destabilizing nature of chronic stress is like a one-two punch to the gut, the head, and just about everywhere else. If you want a fighting chance at balancing your hormones and easing your perimenopause symptoms, you have to learn to manage your stress.

Thankfully, it's not that hard to do with the right food, exercise, and lifestyle habits. I will show you how to simmer down your stress levels using your most powerful tool: your own body.

Superwoman Syndrome

Time and time again I have seen my friends and clients struggle with "superwoman syndrome," a phenomenon publicly decried since at least the 1970s. This term summarizes the societal pressure on a woman to not only perform but excel in all of her careers: her career in the workforce, her career as a mother, her career as a wife, and her career as a friend. Quite frankly, it's impossible to meet this expectation. I am not saying that a woman cannot do all of these things in her life, and do them well—she can—but she cannot do them *perfectly*.

"Perfect" is a tricky little word, an insidious concept that has seeped into fibers of femininity. The perfect superwoman ideal deludes her into stringing a tightrope between her home and her office, over soccer games, parent-teacher conferences, dinner, and presentations at work. It then forces her to walk this hair-thin suspension while carrying a spouse, 2.5 kids, and the dog—and wearing high heels. This superwoman must appear thin, beautiful, graceful, humble, and fun, and do so *effortlessly*. It's impossible to check every box. I can feel my heart beating faster just thinking about it.

The thing about stress is that the body cannot tell the difference between physical and psychological stress. It reacts the same way to both. Whether it's a fight with your child or a fender bender, the exact same physiological process occurs within your body. Superwoman syndrome, and the accompanying physical and psychological strain it creates, is no exception.

Indeed, women seem to be under a disproportionate amount of stress in this day and age. According to the American Psychological Association's 2015 Stress in America survey, women report higher stress levels than men and have consistently done so since the first Stress in America survey in 2007. The APA also found that women consistently report experiencing extreme stress and rising stress levels as well as feeling that they are doing an inadequate job of managing their stress. If you are a woman of color and/or LGBTQ, the APA found that your stress levels are even higher.

While some women learn how to effectively manage their lives, others struggle. They turn to maladaptive coping strategies, such as drinking, overeating, and, increasingly, abusing prescription drugs. In fact, MSNBC published an article in 2010 entitled "Superwoman

Syndrome Fuels Pill-Pop Culture: Overwhelmed Overachievers Turn to Prescription Drugs for an Edge." The article reports the growing issue of high-achieving woman, like lawyers and psychologists, who use prescriptions drugs to keep up and to get ahead. Add on perimenopause, and I think it can take a superwoman just to get out of bed in the morning.

There's a better way to handle stress and balance a full, enriching lifestyle while managing perimenopause symptoms. Going against the superwoman rhetoric, you must put yourself first, taking steps to reduce your stress so that you can show up as a better version of yourself in all areas of your life. Give yourself permission to be imperfect, to make mistakes, to ask for help, and to actually find pleasure in your life. The best first step you can take in reducing stress is to understand how it affects your body. You need to know what's at stake.

Running on Fumes

Think of your body as a luxury vehicle—an artfully constructed machine. You spend your life taxing this amazing machinery as you speed from place to place, from responsibility to responsibility, and from challenge to challenge. All of this exertion creates stress in your body, and that's not necessarily a bad thing. Stress is your body's natural reaction to a stressor—anything that is perceived as a threat to your physical or emotional homeostasis (the maintenance of normal bodily processes within a fixed range). Stressors are intensified by unpredictability, a feeling of a lack of control, and an absence of an outlet for the stress.

Your body's stress response evolved with the primal goal of allowing you to escape predators and other high-stakes situations. Today, it keeps the engines of your luxury vehicle revved and all systems on alert in order to tackle the obstacles in your life. However, nobody with even the most basic knowledge of automobiles would expect their car to stay running forever, the engine still revving even while the vehicle sits in the garage overnight. Stress becomes a problem when it doesn't allow your body to take the keys out of your hormonal ignition, when it forces your body to run on fumes.

Your body has only so many resources it can devote to living in a stressful situation before it begins to deteriorate. Let's take a look to see what those long days filled with traffic, crying kids, and unsympathetic bosses are actually doing to it.

The autonomic nervous system, which is part of the peripheral nervous system, controls your body's involuntary functions and responses, such as breathing, digestion, and, yes, the stress response. The autonomic nervous system consists of two parts: the sympathetic and the parasympathetic nervous systems.

In a short-term, acutely stressful situation, your sympathetic nervous system is activated. Your brain sends messages via your spinal cord and your endocrine system to initiate the fight-or-flight response, preparing your body for the rigorous activity needed to avoid an imminent threat. Remember, stress is all about utilizing your resources in order to survive an intense environmental circumstance.

When in this state, stress hormones like adrenaline (epinephrine), cortisol (cortisone, hydrocortisone), and norepinephrine (noradrenaline) are released throughout your body. Your heart rate and blood pressure increase, and all actions deemed nonessential to immediate survival, such as digestion and tissue repair, are depressed in order for your body to focus all its energy on surviving the immediate danger.

After the danger disappears, the parasympathetic nervous system returns your body to rest as your heart rate decreases, and digestion and other previously hindered functions speed back up. You no longer need to be turned on, so to speak, because there is not a current threat to your survival. This is a healthy stress response functioning as nature intended it to.

But what happens when your body feels constantly under attack; when you're anxious, overworked, and exhausted; when your stress response stays on high alert? In chronically stressful situations, the parasympathetic nervous system does not kick in to relax your body into a state where it can rest and perform critical functions, such as tissue repair and menstruation. Dramatic hormonal and other disruptions continue to occur, possibly to the point of damaging your body. Some of these disruptions affect your hormones.

> REPRODUCTIVE HORMONES: Have you ever missed your
> period because you were stressed out? Interference with
> reproductive hormones due to stress can lead to a disruption
> of the menstrual cycle. Recall from chapter 7 that this can

interrupt the release of progesterone—a vital hormone, especially for female health, that counterbalances estrogen and creates perimenopause symptoms when deficient. Testosterone levels drop too, leading to problems in both sexes, including decreased libido, muscle loss, slowed metabolism, weakened bones, and increased anxiety and depression.

THYROID HORMONE: Stress causes the thyroid, usually stimulated by the adrenal glands to produce hormones, to produce less thyroid hormone, which can lead to thyroid dysfunction, such as hyperthyroidism and hypothyroidism (more about this in chapter 10).

INSULIN: When the body is stressed, insulin levels decrease and cells become less responsive to its actions, raising blood sugar levels and, over time, contributing to insulin resistance.

CATECHOLAMINES: Catecholamines are a class of hormones that includes dopamine, adrenaline, and norepinephrine. Stress increases catecholamine levels, which in turn elevates heart rate, slows digestion, and increases water retention and blood pressure.

Of the many other hormones equally responsive to stress, the most important is cortisol. The hypothalamic-pituitary-adrenal axis triggers the adrenal glands to release this hormone that is so integral to how stress and your body function. Adrenaline is the acute stress hormone, and cortisol is the chronic stress hormone. While both are crucial parts of the stress response, when your body encounters prolonged stress, cortisol takes center stage. And here is where the problem lies: not only are many of your bodily functions repressed during chronic stress, but prolonged exposure to cortisol also ravages the body.

7 PERI ZAPPER
Stress Reliever

Stress makes cortisol levels go out of whack. This results in the digestive slowdown, and even the dreaded belly fat. So coping and managing stress will help your waistline and your hormones in the long run.

Cortisol

Cortisol in itself, like stress, is not a bad thing. As the primary stress hormone, it acts as somewhat of a director of other hormones in the body. It cues a variety of essential processes and gives you the energy to get up and go when you need to. Its goal is to prepare and replenish the body.

Sounds great, right? But with cortisol it is easy to have too much of a good thing. When you begin to notice fatigue setting in, a heightened sensitivity to stressors, and increased emotional reactivity, your cortisol red flags should start to go up.

You exist on a cortisol rhythm. It normally operates on a curve, spiking in the morning in order to help you wake up and then lulling in the evening to allow you to fall asleep. Cortisol works in tandem with melatonin, the sleep hormone. As cortisol levels rise, melatonin levels fall, and vice versa. Stress not only creates an excess of cortisol but also disrupts your cortisol rhythm. When your cortisol rhythm is disrupted, so is your sleep. This leaves you with that all too familiar feeling of lying in bed at night, exhausted, but with eyes wide open. It can cause energy crashes during the day and awakenings in the middle of the night.

Cortisol's impact extends far beyond a bad night's sleep. It is a glucocorticoid, a type of corticosteroid hormone that affects the metabolism of sugar. Remember that during times of stress your body thinks that it needs to use all of its resources to avoid some impending doom. Cortisol is one of the main hormones that allows for this mass utilization of your body's stockpiles.

What do you need to run from a predator? Energy—and fast. Accordingly, cortisol causes the release of glucose into the bloodstream in anticipation of a large energy exertion in that very moment. Cortisol also releases amino acids to prepare to repair damaged tissue. To access glucose and amino acids, cortisol breaks down fatty acids, glycogen, and muscle tissue, which can eventually lead to muscle deterioration.

However, in the modern world, a threat is more likely to be an email on a static computer screen rather than a predator encountered in the forest. You do not need the same amount of energy for vigorous typing as you do for a fistfight with a bear. So instead of using up all the sugar that cortisol has just released, the body stores it in the bloodstream.

Recall from our discussion of carbohydrates what happens to excess sugar in the bloodstream: it turns to fat. Furthermore, cortisol actually stops the secretion of insulin in order to increase the amount of sugar in your blood. If some insulin does manage to get secreted, cortisol makes cells unreceptive to this blood sugar hormone, thus contributing to insulin resistance. Not only do you gain weight, but now you have all the hormonal disruptions of erratic blood sugar levels and high stress working together to overwhelm your system.

As a result, your appetite increases. To add insult to injury, sugary, high-carb foods also release endorphins that work to minimize the stress response, making your body crave them even more. You feel anxiety—nervous energy trapped in your body with nowhere to put it. I know this feeling all too well, and it drives me up the wall!

On top of increasing blood sugar, cortisol is the premier fat storage hormone. I know, I did just say that cortisol breaks down fat, but in the long run, you will definitely gain more than you lose, and not in a good way. In fact, elevated cortisol is associated with obesity, depression, and food addiction. In its love affair with fat, cortisol activates enzymes to store fat when it comes into contact with any and all fat cells. Abdominal fat has four times more cortisol receptors than any other fat cells in the body and can even secrete its own cortisol, making stress a particularly pointed curator of belly fat. Indeed, abdominal fat and a high waist-to-hip ratio are telltale signs of cortisol imbalance. Cortisol increases belly fat not only superficially but also on a deeper level, promoting visceral fat, the kind that surrounds the organs. Visceral fat releases inflammatory proteins and hormones that can damage the body, increasing the risk of chronic disease, inflammation, and mortality.

An expanding gut might be accompanied by a shrinking brain when under chronic stress. Are you finding yourself more forgetful? It might not be your age catching up with you. The brain uses a region called the hippocampus to learn and to process and store memories. This seahorse-shaped structure happens to have a lot of cortisol receptors that can get overwhelmed when cortisol levels surge for extended periods of time. The result: the brain literally shrinks—the hippocampus atrophies, and memory and learning are damaged. Bad news for stressful exam time.

The worst part about stress and perimenopause is that perimenopause and excess cortisol exacerbate each other. Chronic stress in itself already leads to adrenal exhaustion, as the gland is constantly triggered to produce stress hormones. However, during perimenopause, the adrenal glands have to pick up the hormonal slack and compensate for lowering estrogen levels by producing estrogen themselves. This means cortisol's main regulator is distracted, and cortisol rhythms can be disrupted even in someone who has healthy stress levels. Furthermore, adrenal exhaustion can be connected to almost every hormonal problem a person experiences. Excess cortisol, in turn, intensifies other unpleasant symptoms of perimenopause, such as weight gain, bone loss, anxiety, depression, and memory loss.

#8 PERI ZAPPER
Adrenal Refresher

Healthy adrenals are important for everyone in our fast-moving world, but they're especially important during perimenopause. As the backup system for the reproductive organs, your adrenals are designed to step in and assist with the body's declining hormonal output. So at this stage in life, it's as critical as ever to consume a wide spectrum of vitamins, minerals, and adaptogens on a daily basis.

DHEA and Pregnenolone

The adrenal cortex makes small amounts of all the sex hormones but makes large amounts of dehydroepiandrosterone (DHEA) in both men and women. DHEA is intimately tied to the metabolic processes that yield progesterone, estrogen, testosterone, and cortisol. Cholesterol is the originating molecule for all these compounds, including pregnenolone (the grandmother of corticosteroid hormones) and DHEA (the mother of corticosteroid hormones).

Taking non-prescription doses of DHEA or pregnenolone is claimed to confer all kinds of health benefits on users, including protection against aging, burning muscle pain, depression, fatigue, stress, diabetes, lupus, and cancer. The problem with taking DHEA and pregnenolone is that they are hormones involved in little-known biochemical interactions, which means that each has a wealth of potential side effects. The side effects that may be associated with long-term use of DHEA or pregnenolone are simply not known. There have already been complaints from women taking DHEA of growth of facial hair and deepening of the voice. But the most serious potential side effect is the stimulation of breast cancer, because DHEA can raise estrogen levels. Many perimenopausal women are too estrogen dominant to begin with, as I have pointed out time and again.

My suggestion is that, instead of taking possibly dangerous hormones, you should boost the adrenal glands—which secrete these hormones—with adrenal glandulars. However, if you are still considering taking straight DHEA, ask your doctor for the following blood tests: DHEA, DHEAS, and serum tests of free testosterone and estradiol. In this way, you and your physician can monitor your baseline levels and retest to adjust the dosage at regular intervals. A state-of-the-art twenty-four-hour urine test is now available for DHEA and its metabolites (see Resources).

Be the Zebra

Fortunately, there are a multitude of other ways to cope with stress. As you have seen, stress is a bodily reaction, so it follows that you can also use the body to counteract stress—especially psychological stress, the most prevalent kind in today's developed world.

In his classic book *Why Zebra's Don't Get Ulcers,* Stanford University professor Robert Sapolsky explains that zebras don't get ulcers because they use their stress response the way it is meant to be used. A zebra experiences a threat that endangers its life, like encountering a lion, the zebra either escapes the lion or is caught, and then the zebra returns to a resting state—or dies.

In the modern world, stress is not so straightforward. You have already seen the stressful impact of omnipresent forces, like the superwoman syndrome. These cultural, societal, and psychological stressors are not immediately life-threatening. Instead, these survivable stressors persist through daily life, like one lion after another. If the stressors won't go away, then you must learn, within biological reason, how to calm and control your stress response.

Stress-Spiking Foods

Your dietary choices can have a drastic impact on your stress levels. On the most basic level, the foods you eat can stress out your body. Foods like sugar and gluten will act as chemical stressors, inciting a type of systemic inflammation that raises cortisol levels. Food allergies and sensitivities, inflammatory in their own right, will cause the exact same reaction. Remember, no matter where it comes from, stress is stress, and your body has only one response to it—fight or flight.

Caffeine is a particularly bad, stress-boosting offender. It takes only 15 ounces of coffee to raise your adrenaline level by more than 200 percent. Caffeine also promotes norepinephrine production, a catecholamine that is one of the main stress hormones; it targets your nervous system and brain. Even worse, caffeine prevents cortisol reduction and decreases insulin sensitivity. Chugging around three cups of coffee a day could cause your serum cortisol to stay at high levels eighteen out of every twenty-four hours instead of just the couple of hours the body is designed to handle. In fact, caffeine actually reduces your threshold for stress so that you aren't able to handle it as well. You may find coffee relaxing, but your body sure doesn't.

Easy Eating

Reducing stress is not all about avoiding the bad foods. Your diet is your friend, and you can use it to improve your ability to cope with stress. Since fat makes up 60 percent of the brain and every single cell membrane, plus it has vital hormone-regulating properties, fat is your eating ticket to the easy life—well, *easier* life.

For this reason, I highly recommend omega-3 fats as sexy, slimming stress busters. According to the National Institutes of Health, omega-3s help to balance stress hormone levels and to provide direct weight loss benefits. They can be supplied by fatty fish and fish oil, camelina oil, and walnuts and walnut oil.

The omega-derived EPA and DHA fats from fatty fish, like wild-caught salmon, sardines, and anchovies, are major players in regulating emotions and mood, and in warding off depression. These fats have been shown in a number of clinical studies to help reduce aggression and hostility too. They can fortify your system so you can mentally handle and cope with stress more efficiently, minimizing the damage created by elevated levels of cortisol. Fish oil also increases insulin sensitivity so your body can better handle otherwise disruptive blood sugar spikes. The combination of increased insulin sensitivity and decreased cortisol levels makes fish oil an unparalleled aid in lowering stress levels and losing weight. In fact, a study published in the *Journal of the International Society of Sports Nutrition* showed that over the course of six weeks, healthy subjects who had 2,400 milligrams of fish oil per day effectively decreased their cortisol levels in the morning and had leaner bodies. The ocean really is good for the soul!

Camelina oil—derived from the seeds of wild flax, or false flax—is a rich source of plant-based omega-3 ALA. It also contains an amazingly high amount of stable monounsaturated fatty acids (omega-7s) as well as vitamin E, which makes it a very beneficial oil for medium-heat cooking. Due to its high antioxidant content, camelina oil is known as the "better" flax.

ALA-rich walnuts and walnut oil, however, unlike fish or fish oils, are rich in trace minerals like calcium, copper, manganese, selenium, and zinc. Walnuts and walnut oil also pack a serious dose of vitamins B1, B2, B3, and E—all notable stress relievers that soothe the nervous system. Walnuts are also one of the richest natural sources of the hormone melatonin—second only to tart cherries. Melatonin fluctuates in opposition to cortisol to control the sleep–wake cycle. Typically, cortisol peaks in the morning to wake you up, which is when melatonin reaches its lowest point. Likewise, melatonin typically peaks at night to lull you to sleep while your cortisol dips to its lowest level.

Eating foods rich in omega-3 right before bed—like a couple of walnuts or some walnut oil in a smoothie—will come in very handy when you consider that just one night of poor sleep can raise cortisol by 45 percent. This is imperative, as sleep and other lifestyle factors are decisive in your stress level.

During times of high stress, it is also important to eat healthy carbohydrates (along with sexy, slimming fats and protein) because they help reduce cortisol levels. No, this does not mean eat a whole cake. Remember that sugar and other inflammatory foods like glutenous grains increase stress in the body. Instead, opt for whole-food carb sources, such as oatmeal, quinoa, peas, sweet potatoes, squash, and beets. If you have high cortisol levels, then cycle your carbs throughout the day to help mimic your natural cortisol rhythm. This means eating the smallest amount of carbs at breakfast when cortisol levels peak and the largest amount of carbs at dinner, when cortisol levels should be on their way down.

Supplements can also take the biological edge off stress. The M 'n' M Peri Zapper #3 will help modulate cortisol, particularly the B complex and C vitamins. Be sure to take your last portion of magnesium before bed, which will ease you to sleep. You can add in omega-3s as well, with fish oil or flaxseed oil.

Easy Sleeping

For some reason people in the United States don't like to sleep, or if they do, they certainly don't act like it. A poll conducted by Gallup in 2013 showed that 40 percent of us get less than six hours of sleep per night. Moreover, Gallup has consistently reported this number since 1990. The average amount of sleep we get falls short as well, coming in at around 6.8 hours since 1990. As the poll numbers show, almost half the country's population is putting undue stress on their body and functioning at a suboptimal level.

This addiction to wakefulness is a walking nightmare. When you don't get enough sleep, you put your body under stress, depriving it of its critical time to repair tissue, reset hormones, and consolidate memories. During perimenopause, sleep is particularly important to give a solid foundation to hormones that naturally want to go over the edge.

One of the main purposes of the cortisol curve and the curve of its sister, melatonin, as you now know, is to control the sleep–wake cycle. For this reason, getting enough sleep is absolutely foundational to restoring healthy cortisol rhythms and reducing stress. In only two weeks, reducing your shut-eye from eight hours to six hours has significant repercussions on your cortisol curve. It can also increase low-grade, chronic inflammation and decrease insulin sensitivity as well as put you at a higher risk for all the conditions associated with these factors, such as obesity, type 2 diabetes, and heart disease.

How much sleep do you typically get in a night? If the answer is less than eight hours, then it's time to make some changes, especially in the onset of stressful perimenopause. Experts say you need seven to eight hours to maintain healthy functioning and save yourself from stress—but I say push for eight if you can. To some of you, it may sound inconvenient to find the time to get *eight hours* of sleep. But I assure you, you can do it. Even if you aren't immediately falling asleep in your first attempts at an earlier bedtime, keep trying. You're still giving your body the opportunity to rest, relax, and restore its normal rhythms.

Here are my best sleep tips to help you get the shut-eye you need:

- TURN OFF ELECTRONICS AT LEAST ONE HOUR BEFORE BEDTIME: Our beloved devices that we can't live without emit a type of light called blue light, which mimics daylight. Your body cannot tell the difference between the kind of blue light you see outside at noon and the kind you see from your device at midnight—and it reacts to both the same way, reducing the sleep hormone melatonin.

- CREATE A SLEEP-PROMOTING ENVIRONMENT: Sleep in a quiet, dark, cool room—ideally between 62 and 70°F—that is absent of electronic devices. A warm temperature impedes sleep and causes restlessness, and electronics emit electromagnetic radiation (electropollution) that can stress the adrenals, creating intermittent awakenings and fluctuating cortisol levels. Use a fan or air conditioner to keep you cool and comfortable, and disable all wireless devices within three hundred feet of the bedroom, if possible.

- SLEEP ON A SCHEDULE: Try going to bed at the same time every night and waking up with the sunrise. I recommend going to bed around 10 p.m. This will mimic your natural cortisol rhythm as closely as possible. Getting an hour of morning sunlight, or using extremely bright lights in the morning, could help with falling asleep at night.

- TAKE A WARM BATH: Researchers suggest that taking a fifteen-minute bath of 105°F approximately ninety minutes before going to bed is helpful. The rise in body temperature, followed by the decline in the core temperature, signals the body that it's bedtime. Add some lavender or chamomile essential oil to the bath to enhance your relaxation.

- AVOID EATING OR EXERCISING IN THE TWO HOURS BEFORE BEDTIME: Both of these things can cause hormonal disruptions, namely with cortisol and insulin, that interfere with sleep.

- CREATE A NIGHTTIME ROUTINE: Practicing a specific bedtime ritual will establish a set behavior pattern that cues your brain to relax and go to sleep. I strongly encourage you to incorporate relaxation techniques into this routine. Take a warm bath, meditate, or journal to reduce sleep-sabotaging anxiety and quiet your mind and body.

- BE MINDFUL OF NAPS: Try not to nap after 4 p.m. If you do need a quick reenergizer, try a twenty- to thirty-minute nap in the middle of the day.

Easy Exercising

As you know, the entire purpose of the stress response is to prepare your body for vigorous activity. One of the most detrimental parts of stress in this day and age is the absence of activity that would use up all the resources your body has prepared during its fight-or-flight responses. To remedy stress, add back in that exertion. That's why exercise is one of your most powerful stress-busting tools.

While exercise increases stress and raises cortisol in the moment, it will teach your body to better handle stress, and it reduces cortisol in the long run. It also produces calming, pleasurable types of neurotransmitters, such as endorphins, serotonin, and dopamine. Yes, dopamine is one of the catecholamines I implicated in the stress response earlier, but its primary function is to produce pleasurable feelings, like it does with exercise. In fact, a Duke University study found that exercising for thirty minutes a day, three to four times per week, can be as effective as an antidepressant medication for treating depression and anxiety.

Remember, exercise is a type of controlled stress. If excessive stress is dangerous, that means overexercising is too. It is important to watch the intensity of your exercise routine, following the prescription in the previous chapter. Overexercising can have the exact opposite of the desired effect, increasing stress and creating the real potential for weight gain, injury, illness, and the hormonal destabilization that comes with stress. Do not participate in continuous strenuous exercise for more than two hours.

Easy Breathing

Take a deep breath. Good. You just took a positive step toward stress reduction.

Stress is either physical or psychological. Period. As a result, you can use your psychology and your physiology to reduce stress. The most important tool you have—besides sleep and exercise—that addresses both of these things is meditation. No, not medication, *meditation*. In truth, the strongest drug you have to stop the stress response in its tracks is your own breath. The trick is to use logic to guide your brain and body into a relaxed state so the parasympathetic nervous system can do its job.

In an actual life-or-death situation in which you would have to take measures to ensure your own survival, you would breathe rapidly in order to prepare for a physical challenge—not deeply. This is the concept that meditation uses to its advantage. By taking deep breaths, you send a signal to your brain that you are not in danger and that you do not need the full arsenal of your fight-or-flight response to be deployed or your body to be on high alert.

Studies have shown that meditation, like stress, changes the brain, but in a good way. In fact, you can almost think of this relaxation technique as stress's inverse. Remember that stress can shrink the hippocampus? A study out of Harvard University found that meditation has the opposite effect, increasing cortical thickness in the hippocampus after eight weeks of mindfulness-based stress reduction. The same study also found a decrease in the brain cell volume of the amygdala. The amygdala is integral to emotions (especially fear) and emotional memory, and it is the first part of the brain to perceive a threat or stressor. Furthermore, meditators literally maintain their minds better than non-meditators as they age. A study from the University of California at Los Angeles found that meditators had increased gray matter volume in multiple regions throughout their brains. Meditation has also been found to improve immune function, feelings of well-being, attention, and concentration.

During perimenopause, meditation can help you build a better body and a brain that is more centered and prepared to take on the challenges of this hectic hormonal time. There are plenty of apps, podcasts, and online videos that will guide you through meditation, such as the popular Headspace. You can also find plenty of books on the topic if you want to take your practice to the next level. For now, try this mindfulness meditation exercise:

> Set a timer for a desired amount of meditation time. For this initial exercise, start with five minutes.
>
> Sit or lie down in a comfortable position. Your eyes can remain closed or open.
>
> Begin to breathe deeply, at a comfortable, slow pace.
>
> Your mind will wander, and that's okay. When thoughts pass through your mind, do not judge them, do not engage with them. Instead, gently return your attention back to your breathing.
>
> Continue this way for five minutes. Eventually increase your time up to ten minutes, gradually or not, as you feel ready.

Easy Itinerary

One of the biggest psychological stressors we face today is our schedule. Women, especially superwomen, keep themselves darting from place to place, chasing after items on to-do lists as long as the rolls of toilet paper they forgot to pick up from the store. If you want to do it all, you have to learn to balance it all, but don't be afraid to ask for help. In reality, by not asking for help, you are taking away from yourself and, by proxy, everything you do.

Delegate to drive out stress! Delegate appropriate responsibilities to those around you. Your spouse, a friend, or even your older children can help with the kids and dinner. Delegate your time intentionally, carving out time for work, family, and "me" time. Treat each time period like a job, a commitment you cannot avoid. When it is time to work, work your butt off. When it is time to be with your family, truly be there with them, active and engaged. When it is "me" time, be present with yourself, and do something that makes you happy. I recommend using some kind of planner to help you implement a successful structure in your life. I especially like the Passion Planner and Bullet Journal systems, as they provide a built-in structure for achieving your goals.

In a *Huffington Post* article, my new friend Rachel Feldman—health coach, business owner, and mom—wrote about how to "wear the superwoman cape with grace." I just love this article. I particularly like her mandate to superwomen everywhere to give themselves "permission to live." By doing so, Feldman said, "you're making it a point to put as much effort into your personal life as you do your professional life. Doing so will make you a healthier and happier mom, wife, and, of course, business owner."

Feldman also advocated for "outsourcing" your life—essentially, delegating. If you are able to, she suggested, hire a housekeeper or order a delivery dinner, to create more space in your day that would have otherwise been dedicated to completing those tasks yourself. If hiring extra help is not possible for you, Feldman pointed out, you have friends and family who may be happy to support you and help out the superwoman in their life. She also recommended using this same strategy for business, utilizing different apps and employees to accomplish tasks.

For the professional perimenopause women, Feldman recommended a few productivity apps with which you can "outsource" a number of tasks and free up more of your time:

> 17HATS: "An all-in-one app that lets you manage your projects, build quotes, capture leads, sign contracts, create invoices, handle finances, and basically do everything else you need to do," Feldman said in the *Huffington Post* article.

> TEAMWORK: "This is a robust project management platform that is key for managing my teams and projects," Feldman said. "I create to-do lists for my team, create milestones, assign tasks, and collaborate on projects via Teamwork."

> TIMETRADE: "TimeTrade is an online appointment scheduling software, which is a critical component to my business because it allows my coaching clients to book easily time to speak with

me based on the availability I've inputted," Feldman described in the article. "This is a huge time saver and money saver for any business."

SOCIAL MEDIA MANAGEMENT: Feldman suggested installing all of your business's social media apps on your phone and linking them so a post on any one platform pushes to the others as well. To schedule and plan social media posts ahead of time, Feldman suggested Edgar, Buffer, or Hootsuite.

According to Feldman, a business owner's most valuable asset is her time, and I think this applies to life owners too. I want you to sit down and think about what is worth spending your time on. In the end, your life is a series of consecutive minutes. What do you want to give them to?

Easy Emotions

Due to the intimately psychological nature of modern stress, you need to make sure you take care of your mental and emotional life if you want a fighting chance at stopping your fight-or-flight response. Along with proper diet, sleep, exercise, and meditation, there are a few more commonsense lifestyle adaptations you can make to prioritize your well-being and say sayonara to stress.

For women in particular, having a strong social network protects against and improves stress. A landmark study from UCLA proves that a unique friendship forms between women. The researchers demonstrated that women who are under stress produce brain chemicals, namely oxytocin, that open them up to making and maintaining friendships with other women. Oxytocin, the bonding hormone, actually mitigates the stress response and prompts women to "tend and befriend"—meaning, tend to children and befriend other women. Men do not have the same response and tend to isolate more when stressed.

Friendships and close relationships also provide a forum through which you can safely talk about and process your psychological stress. It's great to be around people you care about, but to maximize your stress reduction, you need to share whatever feelings and emotions you have tucked up in your busy mind. The effort of simply trying to seem okay when you really want to break down is stressful in itself. Go ahead, superwoman, land on the ground, and be real with the people you love.

A more private way to process your emotions is to journal—a practice I highly recommend. Journaling can help you develop a clearer image of yourself, your patterns, and your motivations. You can use it as a place to vent, analyze, create, or be silly, free from any and all judgment. Try this exercise, called a brain dump: Find a journal, notebook, or four pieces of paper and start writing. Do not stop writing until four pages are filled. Do not pay attention to grammar or the quality of the writing; just write whatever comes to mind. There is nothing too unimportant; just write openly and honestly. After you have filled four pages, see what you have discovered about yourself.

Sometimes doing everything right is not enough. If you feel like you cannot get ahead of your stress, depression, anxiety, anger, relationship problems, or other emotions, seek out a therapist. There is absolutely nothing to be ashamed about in asking for professional help. Perimenopause especially—as life in general—brings with it emotional ups and downs. So I always remind myself of one of the most insightful pieces of advice I ever heard, from Leon C. Megginson: "It is not the strongest or the most intelligent who will survive but those who can best manage change."

10.

Taming the Thyroid

Boost Metabolism, Fight Fatigue, Relieve Depression

Addressing thyroid issues is critical because so many thyroid symptoms masquerade as perimenopause. In fact, this tiny butterfly-shaped gland in your neck has a huge impact on absolutely every aspect of your health. Besides regulating body temperature and driving metabolism, this mighty gland supports the immune system, the nervous system, and the intestines. It influences the brain, muscles, heart, gallbladder, and liver. Thyroid hormones help strengthen hair, nails, and skin, and they support normal bone growth. So it is not surprising that every single cell in your body has thyroid hormone receptor sites.

Many perimenopausal women exhibit symptoms of hypothyroidism even if their thyroid levels are normal. The late Dr. John Lee, who literally wrote the books on women's hormones, theorized that too much estrogen and too little progesterone could be the cause. Boosting your progesterone levels through the use of natural progesterone cream often normalizes thyroid activity without any other treatment.

The American Thyroid Association states that one in eight women will develop a thyroid disorder, and women are five to eight times more likely than men to develop thyroid problems. It is also estimated that thirty million Americans exhibit some type of thyroid disease. I suspect that number is higher—much higher. Too frequently the signs of a malfunctioning thyroid go unrecognized and ignored, as women assume their symptoms are just a normal part of getting older.

You probably already know that hypothyroidism can cause weight gain, cold hands and feet, and extreme tiredness. But thyroid conditions can cause a much wider array of seemingly unrelated symptoms that you perhaps never considered:

- Aching wrists, arms, and hands
- Brain fog
- Brittle nails
- Coarse voice
- Constipation
- Decreased blood pressure
- Decreased libido
- Dementia
- Depression
- Difficulty swallowing pills, lump in the throat
- Dry, scaly skin
- Fluid retention
- Hot flashes
- Inability to concentrate
- Inappropriate hair growth
- Increased cholesterol
- Infertility
- Insomnia
- Irritability
- Loss of appetite
- Menstrual irregularities
- Muscle stiffness

- Muscle weakness and cramping
- Poor eyebrow growth (especially the outer one-third of the brow)
- Premature graying of hair
- Swelling around the eyes

Even subclinical levels of thyroid problems can have unwanted effects, such as increased risk for heart disease and Alzheimer's.

Thyroid 101

A healthy thyroid produces hormones in just the right amounts, primarily thyroxine (T4) and triiodothyronine (T3). The number after the *T* denotes the amount of iodine in the hormone's molecular structure. How much of these hormones your body produces depends on the complex interaction between your body, your hypothalamus, and your pituitary. You may remember the hypothalamus and the pituitary gland from the previous chapter when I talked about the hypothalamic-pituitary-adrenal axis and the stress response. This time, we are looking at the thyroid, not the adrenal glands.

In response to feedback from your body, the hypothalamus (a part of your brain) instructs the pituitary gland (the master gland of the endocrine system) to produce more or less thyroid-stimulating hormone (TSH). TSH does exactly what its name implies: it stimulates the thyroid to produce hormones. A combination of the amount of iodine and TSH determines the type and amount of hormone your thyroid produces. That hormone is then deployed into your body and gives every single cell direction on how much oxygen and nutrients to consume. In other words, T3 and T4 instruct cells whether to increase or decrease your metabolism.

You can often trace the source of hypothyroidism to a nutrient disruption (especially iodine) or to an autoimmune disease. In the case of an autoimmune disorder, it means the body is somehow "attacking" its own thyroid tissue, which is primarily an immune problem, not a thyroid problem. The most common of these autoimmune diseases is Hashimoto's thyroiditis.

Interestingly, the group of people most likely to develop Graves' disease—another autoimmune disease that affects the thyroid—are women in perimenopause. Unlike Hashimoto's, Graves' disease causes hyperthyroidism, not hypothyroidism. Regardless, the overstimulation inherent in Graves' disease can exhaust the thyroid and ultimately lead to hypothyroidism.

Diagnosis

Thyroid issues typically go undiagnosed, particularly when a doctor relies solely on a standard test of TSH and T4 levels.

Why? The line between a normal and an underactive thyroid is very fine indeed. And many physicians are reluctant to order a complete thyroid panel, relying instead on a single TSH blood test to make their diagnosis.

There are five basic thyroid hormone blood tests in conventional medicine.

- TSH (THYROID-STIMULATING HORMONE): Ordered by nearly all physicians when a thyroid problem is suspected, this test measures the signal between your thyroid and your pituitary gland. If your thyroid is functioning properly, your pituitary sends very little TSH, resulting in a low score. There is not a unanimous agreement on what the ideal "normal range" for TSH is, but I favor a range between 0.3 and 2.5 mIU/L (milli-international units per liter). When your TSH is lower than 0.3 mIU/L, you likely have hyperthyroidism. If it is above 2.5 mIU/L, you likely have hypothyroidism. Unfortunately, TSH is the only test that many physicians order when diagnosing thyroid disorders. Relying solely on this test has resulted in many cases of hypothyroidism going untreated.

- T4 (THYROXINE): Of the two thyroid hormones, T4 is the less active one. Your thyroid generates significantly more T4 than T3, with T4 generally making up about 80 percent of the thyroid's output. As a result, your body normally has a "reserve" of T4 ready to be converted into the more active hormone T3. This conversion of T4 to T3 occurs in the organs of the body, such as the kidneys, liver, and brain. When T3 conversion fails to occur at adequate levels, hypothyroidism results.

The conversion of T4 to T3 can be blocked by many factors, including aging, illness, stress, high consumption of soy, and medications (including hormone replacement therapy). Most doctors are fairly open to ordering a test to check T4 levels along with the TSH test. However, since T4 remains useless unless it converts to T3, a normal T4 test tells only part of the story.

- T3 (TRIIODOTHYRONINE): T3 packs three times the punch of T4 and is responsible for revving up the body's metabolism. Because hypothyroidism can still exist despite normal TSH and T4 tests, be sure to ask your physician to check your T3 levels as well.

- ANTITHYROGLOBULIN AND ANTITHYROPEROXIDASE: Some thyroid conditions are autoimmune in nature. This test measures the number of antibodies your body may be making to attack your own thyroid gland.

- TRH (THYROTROPIN-RELEASING HORMONE): Testing this hormone can identify whether your pituitary is giving your thyroid the right signals. Your physician may consider this test if all your other test results are normal but you continue to have symptoms indicative of thyroid disorders.

Even if your TSH levels are normal, high elevation of three non-thyroid hormones can contribute to low thyroid function and will not show up on standard thyroid tests.

- You haven't forgotten about *cortisol* yet, have you? Elevated cortisol levels can assault thyroid function from nearly every angle. They fatigue the pituitary gland, hurting its ability to produce TSH, so the thyroid is never prompted to produce the correct amount of the hormone. This does not damage the thyroid gland itself, but it creates a rift in pituitary–thyroid communication, which prevents the thyroid from properly responding to the body's needs. An elevated cortisol level and inflammation damage cell membranes, making them unable to convert T4 to T3, and therefore unable to truly use either thyroid hormone. Finally, excess cortisol can cause cells to become resistant to thyroid hormones at the receptor sites, making it so that cells cannot receive appropriate signals from the thyroid.

- High *estrogen* levels can elevate thyroid-binding globulin (TBG), a protein that binds to thyroid hormones and assists them on their journey through the bloodstream. When there is a high concentration of TBG, it means much of the thyroid hormones in the body are bound and unavailable for use by the cells. This creates a shortage of thyroid hormones.

- High *testosterone* levels can lower TBG. This has the opposite effect of high TBG and elevates levels of free (unbound) thyroid hormones in the body. However, like insulin and leptin, cells can become resistant to thyroid hormones if they are overexposed to them. For this reason, low TBG levels actually create *hypo*thyroidism, not, like one might expect, *hyper*thyroidism.

Check for Yourself

Are there ways to confirm a diagnosis of hypothyroidism beyond the conventional lab tests? You bet. Some experts believe that T3 and T4 levels can be measured more accurately by means of urine testing. Because it is a more sensitive test, it may pick up subclinical hypothyroidism that otherwise may be missed.

Dr. Broda O. Barnes, who researched thyroid and other endocrine dysfunctions for more than fifty years, developed the Barnes basal temperature test as an indicator of possible thyroid deficiency. When the thyroid fails, a person's resting temperature measures abnormally low. If you take your temperature first thing in the morning for five mornings and it consistently reads below 97.8°F, you may have low thyroid function. In use since the early 1940s in various forms, this test is simple and very sensitive to minor deficiencies, and you can do it at home. Note that if you are menstruating, begin the test four days after the start of your period. Doing so provides the most accurate results.

Before you go to bed, place a basal body thermometer—one that can measure temperatures between 96 and 99°F—on your bedside table. As soon as you wake up, before getting out of bed and without any mental or physical activity, put the thermometer in your mouth and keep it there for a full three minutes. (You may also place the thermometer in your armpit, but it must be left there for a full ten minutes.) Lie quietly while the thermometer is in place.

After doing this test for five mornings in a row and noting your temperature each day, average the results. The following readings are indicative of thyroid states:

Below 97.8°F	Possible hypothyroid
97.8–98.2°F	Normally functioning thyroid
Above 98.2°F	Hyperthyroid or possible infection

Dr. Barnes recommended natural thyroid preparations. Today, cyclic natural time-release thyroid therapy preparations are available through compounding pharmacies.

Iodine

Iodine deficiency is the most common cause of hypothyroidism. The connection between thyroid function and adequate iodine levels became clear decades ago. As you know, the thyroid gland depends on iodine to make its hormones. If your body lacks an adequate level of iodine, your thyroid gland can't produce those all-important T3 and T4 hormones.

To test—and treat—your iodine levels and thyroid function, try this simple remedy that has been used by naturopathic doctors in Europe for decades:

- Gather a cotton swab and some 2 percent tincture of iodine. (Tincture of iodine may be found at most drugstores and supermarkets. It is usually kept with the first-aid supplies and costs less than two dollars a bottle.)

- Dip the cotton swab in the iodine and paint a silver-dollar-size patch on your abdomen or thigh. You should now see a brownish stain. Make sure you allow it to dry before covering it with clothing.

- Check the stain frequently. The goal, and the sign of a well-functioning thyroid, is for the stain to remain visible for at least twenty-four hours.

- If the stain disappears in less than twenty-four hours, your body is deficient in iodine. Paint another silver-dollar-size area as soon as you notice the first stain has disappeared. For example, if your initial stain disappears in two hours, reapply the iodine at that time.

- Continue applying iodine until the stain is still visible after twenty-four hours. For people with severe iodine deficiencies, this process may take weeks!

Keep in mind that if you are already taking thyroid supplementation, you may need to see your doctor to readjust the dosage. It may be possible to discontinue the supplementation altogether, but this would be a decision between you and your physician.

Now you know how important iodine is to a healthy thyroid gland. But there's even more to the story of iodine. Strong evidence exists that women who are deficient in iodine have a higher risk of developing breast cancer. Statistics show that the Japanese, whose diets are high in iodine, have a very low incidence of iodine-deficiency diseases like goiter, hypothyroidism, and cancers of the reproductive system.

As my friend, colleague, and highly respected nutrition expert Nan Fuchs, Ph.D., advises, getting 150 micrograms of iodine per day is enough to prevent the development of a goiter, but many women benefit from more. Keep in mind that iodine is concentrated in both the thyroid gland and breast tissue. Because women have larger breasts than men, we need more iodine than they do.

Back in the 1960s each slice of store-bought bread contained 150 micrograms of iodine. And the rate of breast cancer was one woman in twenty. Now that iodine has been replaced with bromine, a substance that, like fluoride, competes with iodine and increases the risk of goiters, our rate of breast cancer has jumped to one woman in eight. While correlation does not prove causation, I think there is more to this relationship than a suspicious coincidence.

A groundbreaking study by well-known researcher Dr. Bernard A. Eskin showed that rats developed hypothyroidism when they became deficient in iodine. When rats were given the standard treatment for hypothyroidism—thyroid hormone—their breast tissues responded by growing an excessive number of cells. However, when the rats were treated with extra iodine, this abnormal cell growth ceased. Why? Iodine flips off the switch on estrogen receptors in the breast. So when iodine is deficient, the breast tissues respond abnormally to estrogen, putting a woman at risk for precancerous and cancerous conditions. In my experience, most women need 5 milligrams of iodine for normal breast function.

To consume the minimum amount of iodine, add seafood and other iodine-rich foods to your daily diet. Sea vegetables are your best source of iodine, but do take caution when purchasing them. As I mentioned in chapter 5, do not consume sea vegetables that come from Japan, due to the toxic radiation contamination. I recommend getting your sea veggies from Maine or other parts of the northeastern United States (see Resources).

You may find you need more iodine than you can get from food alone. Some of my clients have done well by taking one to two kelp tablets daily. Others have tried supplements such as Prolamine and Iodoral. However, since iodine supplementation can be tricky, and dangerous if executed incorrectly, I recommend you consult a knowledgeable expert before trying it on your own.

The Bile Connection

You may have never considered bile and what it does for your body, but the connection between hypothyroidism and bile is of serious importance. According to a study conducted at Tampere University Hospital in Finland, hypothyroidism may cause delays in the emptying of the biliary tract. Researchers at the same hospital found that hypothyroidism is seven times more likely in people who experience reduced bile flow.

Bile, also known as gall, is a yellow-greenish liver secretion that helps with the digestion of fats in the small intestine. As we age, the toxins that we encounter on a daily basis build up in our bodies, and they become trapped in our bile, resulting in the bile thickening and no longer flowing freely. Excess estrogen only complicates matters, causing cholesterol levels in bile to rise, which adds to the growing thickness and congestion. To pile on another concern, stress decreases the quantity of bile in the body.

When bile cannot function properly, it cannot effectively break down fats in the digestive process, leaving the body to deposit fat as excess weight rather than utilize it in other ways. This means that you will not receive the multitude of health benefits from all of those sexy, slimming fats because the body cannot metabolize this foundational macronutrient.

Bile also affects hormonal function. A study conducted by researchers that included thyroid specialist Dr. Antonio Bianco showed that people who improved their bile health saw a 53 percent increase in their metabolism. The study also showed that the release of bile triggered the release of an enzyme that converts T4 to T3. As you now know, this conversion is critical to facilitate thyroid functioning. When you have healthy bile, you are well on your way to having healthy thyroid hormones.

Fortunately, you can take effective measures to build healthy bile. The first step is to detox, which will signal the body to thin the bile and get it moving again. You can prompt this detox process by eating plenty of fiber-rich veggies, beginning your day with hot lemon water, and sprinkling 1 tablespoon of non-GMO sunflower or soy lecithin in your smoothies or on your salads.

The next step is to increase bile production by consuming healthy protein at each meal and adding more saturated fat to your diet (coconut oil is a great choice). Whether or not you have a gallbladder, which moderates the release of bile, it's also wise to encourage healthy bile production via supplementation. I recommend Uni Key's Bile Builder (see Resources). This supplement is critical for those without a gallbladder and a helpful anti-bloat tool for anyone.

#9   PERI ZAPPER
Liver and Bile Support

Without quality, free-flowing bile, the body lacks the proper ability to break down fat and transport excess hormones out of the body. This leads to poor estrogen metabolism, hypothyroidism, fatigue, indigestion, constipation, and weight gain—provoking perimenopause-related symptoms. Ensure that you're providing your liver what it needs to produce adequate bile with supplementation of choline, lipase, taurine, ox bile, beet root, and collinsonia root.

Give Up the Gluten

You've already heard me strongly urge you to get the gluten out of your life, and its effect on the thyroid only further proves my point. Studies have shown that gluten intolerance and autoimmune thyroid disease share a nefarious connection.

When it comes to the thyroid, the problem with gluten lies with the structure of its protein gliadin. Remember, a gluten intolerance causes the body to attack any gluten in the body. The molecular structure of gliadin so closely resembles that of thyroid tissue that when the body tries to attack gliadin, it attacks the thyroid too. That's right, gluten literally turns the body against its own thyroid gland. Not only does gluten weaken the intestinal walls, increasing intestinal permeability (see chapter 3), but it manipulates and damages the body that lives on the other side of those walls.

For obvious reasons, if you have a problem with your thyroid, you need to give up gluten—and I mean give it up completely. One Italian study found evidence that gluten continues to affect the body for six months after consumption in individuals with celiac disease. Cutting back on foods containing gluten and cheating just "once in a while" won't cut it.

For anyone with celiac disease and gluten intolerance, non-glutenous grains like rice, corn, and oats can still resemble gluten enough to trigger a reaction in the body. If you continue to struggle after giving up gluten, these grains might be your problem.

Address Your Stress

As you have already read, chronic stress and the high cortisol levels that come with it are another enemy of thyroid health. Everything you read in the previous chapter about stress reduction applies just as much to thyroid health as it does to whole-body health. After all, the thyroid is one of your chief hormone regulators, and stress is one of your chief hormone disruptors.

In conjunction with stress reduction, I encourage you to explore supplements that nourish your adrenals in order to further support your thyroid. When your adrenal glands are well nourished, your thyroid will be supported too. Adrenal glandulars are supplements made up of actual adrenal gland tissue from animal sources, usually cows or pigs. These supplements can restore and stabilize the often overworked stress glands. They are also more easily discontinued than a synthetic cortisol hormone replacement once the adrenals are functioning normally again. If you are unwilling to consume an animal product, try adaptogenic herbs like ashwagandha.

Fear Fluoride

How many times have you brushed your teeth with fluoride-filled toothpaste? Probably a lot. Dentists and other health experts hail fluoride as a fierce fighter of tooth decay. In fact, fluoride is added to about two-thirds of the water supply in the United States, supposedly to prevent cavities. The CDC included water fluoridation as one of its "Ten Great Public Health Interventions of the 20th Century."

However, just because fluoride purportedly prevents tooth decay does not means it prevents thyroid decay. In 2015, English researchers at the University of Kent published a study in the *Journal of Epidemiology and Community Health* that looked at data from nearly every general medical practice in that country, the largest population ever studied in regards to water fluoridation. They found that individuals who lived in communities with fluoridated water had a 30 percent higher chance of developing hypothyroidism. This amounted to 9 percent more occurrences of hypothyroidism in communities with fluoridated water than communities that did not fluoridate their water.

Fluoride, along with bromide and chlorine, interferes with the thyroid's uptake of iodine, an element necessary to thyroid hormone production. Think of it this way: the more fluoride, the less thyroid hormone produced—hence, hypothyroidism.

Even though topical fluoride, like that in toothpaste (when you don't swallow it), may improve dental health, public water fluoridation has had its critics since its inception. In 2012, researchers at Harvard's School of Public Health, alongside researchers from China and

Denmark, named fluoride as a possible neurotoxin. The researchers reviewed twenty-seven studies from across the globe and found evidence that water fluoridation may lower IQ in children if they are exposed during development. Critics have even cited multiple studies that question the true efficacy of fluoride in the water supply. In places like Japan, the Netherlands, Finland, Cuba, and Canada, the rate of tooth decay actually decreased after discontinuing water fluoridation. Nevertheless, the CDC maintains that current research continues to support the safety and protective benefits of water fluoridation.

I encourage you, alongside avoiding fluoridated water, to be wary of processed food and tea—green tea, in particular—for its high fluoride content. If you drink tea, opt for an herbal tea, like the liver-boosting dandelion root tea. And if you can't kick that green tea habit, try to find a high-quality, pure tea, like matcha, that will likely have little or no fluoride. I also suggest you look into a water filtration system that removes fluoride (more about this in chapter 13).

Befriend Your Intestines

At least 20 percent of thyroid function relies on a healthy amount of beneficial bacteria in the gut. One strain in particular has been found to protect against the toxicity of gliadin, which is so problematic for thyroid health. That strain is *B. lactis BI-04* and comes from the Bifidobacterium family.

You know the benefits of probiotics from foods like yogurt, kefir, and cultured vegetables in boosting gut flora. You can increase your probiotic intake exponentially with a well-balanced probiotic supplement containing a variety of different strains. The right balance of friendly flora will support your thyroid and many other immune-enhancing processes.

And More . . .

There are still more thyroid threats that tamper with its function: Viruses can sabotage your thyroid, especially dental and sinus viruses, as well as the Epstein-Barr virus and general viral overload. Agents such as goitrogens (found in raw cruciferous vegetables, lecithin, and soy), bromine, and chlorine all act in a similar manner to fluoride and interfere with the thyroid's uptake of iodine. In addition, a lack of protein hampers thyroid function.

Sexy, Smart Fats First

While all the sexy, slimming fats will help heal an ailing thyroid, none work quite the same magic as coconut oil. It boosts thyroid efficiency and stakes a claim as the only fat that does not require bile to break it down, letting it bypass the gallbladder. This means it can work its wonders on the thyroid regardless of bile health. Coconut oil also has antiviral properties; it can help fend off viral overload as well as viruses like Epstein-Barr, which specifically targets this crucial hormone-regulating gland.

Get Rid of the Goitrogens

Raw cruciferous vegetables, including brussels sprouts, cabbage, cauliflower, and kale, all contain potential thyroid saboteurs called goitrogens. Fortunately, cooking these otherwise nutritious vegetables neutralizes their thyroid-threatening features. With regards to soy products, only consume fermented GMO-free soy products or GMO-free lecithin, which does not contain the goitrogenic element.

Maximize with Micronutrients

In addition to iodine, the thyroid needs several trace elements in order to maintain normal hormone metabolism. These elements include selenium, zinc, and copper. When I say zinc and copper, I am referring to the same all-important zinc-copper balance I discussed in chapter 6. You need to have these two minerals in balance to have a healthy thyroid. Furthermore, zinc helps boost T3, the more active thyroid hormone, by raising free levels of it in the body and helping to convert T4 to T3. It also lends a helping hand to the pituitary gland, assisting it in producing the correct amount of TSH.

Although zinc and copper are now common knowledge to you, selenium may strike you as more unfamiliar. Selenium plays a role in both immunity and thyroid function. It seems to mitigate iodine toxicity and associated autoimmune disorders as well as aid in the generation of thyroid hormones and the conversion of T4 to T3. Deficiency in this element is not associated with any particular disease but rather causes a hindrance in the processes it supports. You can find selenium in seafood, such as halibut, salmon, scallops, shrimp, and tuna; in land-bound animals, such as chicken, eggs, lamb, and turkey; and, for vegetarians, in cremini and shiitake mushrooms.

There are some other nutrients that are specifically thyroid friendly, and a deficiency in any one of them may result in thyroid dysfunction. The important thyroid-supporting nutrients include the following, with a suggested daily dosage most commonly recommended by nutritional experts:

Nutrient	Dosage
Vitamin A	25,000 IU
Vitamin B2	15 mg
Vitamin B6	25 to 50 mg
Vitamin E	400 IU
Iodine	50 to 150 mcg
Iron	10 to 15 mg
Selenium	100 to 200 mcg
Zinc	20 to 30 mg

11.

Estrogen, Phytoestrogens, and Bioflavonoids

Learning Truth and Balance

I f there was anything you really believed before reading this book, I bet you thought that estrogen levels plummet during the change before the change. The truth is that while during menopause estrogen does decrease, the overall hormonal fluctuations that occur during perimenopause can actually leave you with either too little or *too much* estrogen. This is because for much of perimenopause nutrient deficiencies, a low level of balancing progesterone, and exhausted adrenals with a tired-out thyroid can cause hormonal imbalances and consequent symptoms.

In perimenopause, estrogen (like its sister, progesterone) starts to fluctuate, leaving the classic menopausal symptoms in its wake: hot flashes, night sweats, and tissue dryness. While low estrogen has a far-reaching effect on your metabolism, excess estrogen is the ultimate hormone magnet for sodium and fat. As I mentioned previously, progesterone production slows during perimenopause, causing estrogen dominance. Estrogen dominance is, in part, responsible for perimenopausal symptoms like weight gain, depression, loss of libido, and hair loss.

Yes, perimenopause throws your hormones off balance, but by decoding all your body's distress signals and making some simple diet and lifestyle changes, you can take charge of your perimenopause while speeding up metabolism, overcoming stress, banishing hunger, and dialing back hormonal weight gain. You can manage this without medications like Prozac, sleeping pills, artificial hormones, or anti-anxiety meds, which simply cover up symptoms without fixing the root causes. Regulating estrogen is no different. You may very well not need a drastic medical treatment like hormone replacement therapy. Rather, you can address the underlying imbalances through diet and supplementation, which directly improves progesterone levels and bile efficiency, and eliminates estrogen-like xenoestrogens from your lifestyle that impede your body's hormonal function.

In Defense of Estrogen

I'm afraid I have given estrogen a bad rap in this book so far as I depicted the dirty truth of estrogen dominance. But don't forget the magic that can happen when you have balanced estrogen levels. This powerful hormone helps your libido, complexion, brain, and the rest of your body too.

Many of us have heard both that estrogen improves the health of the heart, blood vessels, bones, brain, uterus, and breasts and that it is implicated in breast cancer, uterine cancer, ovarian cancer, autoimmune diseases, fibroids, asthma, mood swings, and migraines. Researchers find it hard to say where the boundaries of estrogen's powers lie or to untangle single estrogen threads from the whole estrogen tapestry. Moreover, they have had to change much of their previous thinking about this hormone because of some unexpected discoveries about how it controls target cells.

Hormones like estrogen bind with cell receptors to form molecules that go directly to the cell's DNA to issue instructions. It was always assumed that this was a simple on/off process, like a light switch. The process was off when the receptor was empty and on when the hormone filled its receptor. But our bodies are more complicated than that.

Researchers have found that different kinds of estrogen and estrogen-like drugs, upon settling into a receptor, cause the resulting molecule to assume different shapes. The shape of the combined estrogen receptor molecule affects the choice of DNA genes that receive instructions. For example, one shape might affect bone genes, but not breast genes.

Then researchers discovered that estrogen had another receptor—not just one! They called the receptor they had known about the alpha receptor, and the second one the beta receptor. The beta receptor proved to be present in organs that had not previously been thought to be under the influence of estrogen, such as the large and small intestines, kidneys, bladder, and lungs.

Alpha Receptor Dominant	Beta Receptor Dominant
Blood vessels	Blood vessels
Brain and nerves	Bones
Breasts	Brain and nerves
Uterus (women)	Intestines
	Lungs
	Ovaries (women)
	Prostate (men)
	Testes (men)
	Urogenital tract

The discovery of the beta receptor was of immediate clinical importance, because cancer specialists biopsy breast tumors for the presence of estrogen receptors, to see if the cells are likely to be inhibited from growth by estrogen-like drugs. If estrogen receptors are absent, there is no point in using estrogen-like drugs. But present-day biopsies are designed to find only the alpha receptor; so if only beta receptors are present, a false result may be given that no receptors are present, and a possibly life-saving therapy will not be tried.

It is plainly a misconception to think of estrogen only as a female hormone, or even as purely a sex hormone. With estrogen's presence in so many organs, it must be thought of as one of the body's main chemical messengers. While estrogen has long been credited as beneficial for the heart, the presence of both alpha and beta receptors in the linings of blood vessels suggests its direct role in cardiovascular health. Adequate estrogen is also a surprising weight loss catalyst. When you have low estrogen levels, your body cannot generate as much choline, a nutrient that supports healthy weight by bettering the bile and reducing fat on the liver. Without choline, you can end up with a congested liver or fatty liver that cannot produce quality bile or sufficiently detoxify the body, potentially leading to estrogen dominance and a host of other symptoms.

Revisiting Estrogen Dominance

Interestingly, estrogen dominance affects both men and women. However, in males, we refer to this excessive estrogen as aromatization. Aromatization describes a disruption in the male estrogen-testosterone balance, not the estrogen-progesterone balance. It causes similar issues in men as it does in females, including decreased libido and weight gain. Although, unlike with women, the weight gain tends to concentrate in the upper body, not the lower body, and men also can experience hair loss and prostate problems.

In both sexes, estrogen dominance is linked to a tired and toxic liver due to a multitude of liver antagonists: bad fats, normal hormonal changes that occur with aging, processed food, medication, and environmental toxins. Both sexes produce various versions of estrogen that must be kept in hormonal harmony. Estrogen, as we know it, actually arises from estradiol, which breaks down into other types of estrogen, including estrone and estrogen metabolites. This breaking down process helps the body to maintain estrogen balance.

When it comes to breaking down estrogen, the liver gets the job done. The liver is the body's "living filter," taking the brunt of unwanted waste products and cleansing them from the body. One of its hundreds of jobs is to inactivate unneeded estrogen and expel it from the body through the bile, urine, and stool. That's why congested bile and poor digestion can contribute to estrogen dominance. The longer unneeded estrogen stays in the body, the more opportunity it has to make its way back into the system. Poor estrogen metabolism can also lead to breast, endometrial, and cervical cancer.

One type of environmental toxin has an exceptionally evil effect on excess estrogen and the liver. Xenoestrogens are human-made chemicals that act as "estrogen mimics." I will go into more detail about xenoestrogens in chapter 13, but know that they can interfere with normal estrogen function as well as overload the liver as it tries to metabolize these hormonal imposters, forcing the liver to struggle to keep up with the amount of unwanted estrogen it must rid from the body. The result is poor detoxification by the liver, congested bile, and estrogen dominance, all leading to a more toxic body.

Specific foods aid in the metabolism of estrogen, including cooked bok choy, broccoli, brussels sprouts, cabbage, and cauliflower. Diindolylmethane (DIM), found in cruciferous vegetables or in supplement form, helps to normalize estrogen metabolism in the liver. Of course, flaxseed will improve estrogen levels too, as it does most everything related to the hormones!

There also seems to be a link between estrogen and histamine intolerance. Estrogen stimulates histamine, and histamine stimulates estrogen. Histamine is the same protein targeted by those antihistamines you may take during pollen season. Outside of that annoying running nose and itchy eyes, histamines also help get the brain working, regulate stomach acid, and boost libido. Plus, they are necessary for female reproductive processes, such as ovulation. Because of their dual stimulatory effect, some women can improve their estrogen dominance by avoiding high histamine foods, such as red wine, sauerkraut, aged cheeses, vinegar, cured meat, and chocolate. To further reduce histamines, avoid foods you may have a sensitivity to, like gluten and dairy, and supplement with vitamin B6.

Teresa

In her mid-fifties, Teresa was plagued by exhaustion, GI woes, and mood swings. The fatigue was debilitating. It was troubling her relationship with her husband and her grandchildren. When the fatigue cost Teresa, a business owner, an important client, she knew she needed help.

"Despite how tired I was, I wasn't sleeping well," Teresa said. Two years earlier, her primary care provider had prescribed hormone replacement therapy (HRT) to ease her menopause symptoms and improve her sleep. "The prescription helped with my hot flashes and mood swings, but it wasn't helping with the fatigue. I was concerned about the long-term risks of the meds, so I stopped taking them. But I began to feel *worse* as new symptoms like GI problems, brain fog, anxiety, and pain set in. I started to worry something was really wrong."

She left a second visit to her doctor with a prescription for an antidepressant. While her mood improved for a while, she still struggled with her other symptoms. Her intuition told her that nutrition was the answer she was looking for. She tried my Fat Flush program and lost twenty pounds. But she was still exhausted. That's when she called me.

Despite the success of a nutrient-dense diet for weight loss, and because Teresa was still exhausted, I suspected she had a bile deficiency. Her prior HRT use indicated too much estrogen, which can lead to congested bile, and that was likely making her liver sluggish and causing her symptoms.

I asked Teresa to support her liver with a cup of hot water and lemon each morning. I recommended a tablespoon of apple cider vinegar before meals to improve bile flow. She was already familiar with the benefit of a nutrient-dense diet from her experience with my Fat Flush plan, but I reminded her to continue to avoid processed foods and sugar, eat organic meat, keep to only two servings a day of low-glycemic fruit like blueberries and raspberries, and enjoy more green leafy veggies. I also encouraged her to eat beets, which contain betaine, a compound that builds bile. I told her that spices like cayenne, turmeric, and cumin would help to detoxify the liver. I recommended supplements of ox bile and choline to help her liver produce adequate amounts of bile and lecithin to break down fats. Choline is a powerful emulsifying agent, making fats easier to digest, and it's a most outstanding nutrient to remedy a fatty liver.

Six weeks later, Teresa had her energy back and had lost another nine pounds. She is thrilled with the revitalization of her relationships, and she has even started a new business as a personal chef, providing healthful meals to clients.

Phytoestrogens

Phytoestrogens are estrogen-like substances found in plants. These substantially weaker chemicals bind to human estrogen receptors and either block or stimulate the receptors to increase or decrease estrogen levels in accordance with the body's needs. They also act as antioxidants, combating free-radical damage, which can contribute to aging and cancer. Overall, phytoestrogens pacify problematic hormone levels and can help produce a more pleasant person inside and out.

When it comes to perimenopause, you can take advantage of the estrogenic properties of phytoestrogens to alleviate your symptoms without condemning yourself to a regimen of unpleasant synthetic hormones. Phytoestrogens are found in more than three hundred plant foods, including apples, carrots, flaxseeds (especially in the lignans), oats, olives, pomegranate seed oil, soybeans, sunflower seeds, and tea, as well as in herbs, such as dong quai. Eating foods high in phytoestrogens can improve female problems pertaining to low libido, vaginal dryness, hot flashes, and thinness of the vaginal wall as well as improve depression and anxiety. While not a phytoestrogen, black cohosh is a superstar herb for female health. It has been shown to help with vasomotor menopausal symptoms like hot flashes and night sweats, improve sexual function, and stabilize estrogen-related symptoms like depression.

Some particular herbs—not all phytoestrogens—are especially effective in helping women reclaim libido and rediscover sexual pleasure, both of which can get lost during perimenopause:

Ashwagandha	Rhodiola
Black cohosh	Sea buckthorn
Korean red ginseng	Tongkat ali
Maca	

Regardless of how you decide to supplement your dwindling estrogens levels, the key for many of my clients is enhancing estrogen metabolism. The elements that do the most to help your liver break down estrogen include choline, inositol, and methionine. DIM (diindolylmethane), calcium d-glucarate, and sulforaphane (which is found in broccoli sprouts) are well-researched estrogen-metabolizing agents as well.

Maggie

At forty-three, Maggie had three teenage daughters, the oldest of whom was nineteen. She had returned to her career as a chartered accountant when the youngest started school. Her husband and she were happily married, shared a relatively high joint income, and had a lovely home in a neighborhood her family enjoyed.

About a month after her forty-third birthday, acute depression hit Maggie out of nowhere. She had known what it was like to have the blues from time to time and had mourned the deaths of both her beloved parents. This depression was nothing like grieving or having the blues. It hit her so strongly, its impact felt physical as well as emotional. It felt like a giant hand pressing her down, and it came and went unpredictably, and when it went, it was never far away. Over the next three months her depression became so debilitating that she had to take a leave of absence from her accounting firm.

Although she saw a psychologist, she had a hard time relieving her depression through weekly talk therapy alone. She next saw a psychiatrist, who tried out different kinds of antidepressants, none of which made her feel much better. Maggie stopped seeing her psychiatrist when she felt the side effects of the medication, like weight gain and fatigue, did not justify any benefit she received from the daily pills.

One evening Maggie was lying on her bed with the lights out and the door closed, feeling bad and increasingly desperate, when her eldest daughter knocked on the door and came in. Without any explanation, she handed her mother a bottle of black cohosh pills and a glass of water. Maggie, surprised at her blind trust in her daughter, swallowed two pills, and her daughter left the room.

The next day, Maggie felt a little better. The depression wasn't gone, but she felt motivated to get out of bed and eat a proper breakfast in the kitchen with her family for the first time in months. She didn't feel spritely, but this was an improvement over her usual routine of eating toaster pastries in bed. She asked her daughter about the pills, but the nineteen-year-old was evasive. She said that a friend had given them to her. Finally, Maggie discovered that black cohosh was an herb for perimenopause.

"I think you feel bad because of your hormones," her daughter said, adding defensively, "My friends think so too."

Although her daughter's concern troubled her, Maggie couldn't help smiling at the thought of the serious conversations that her now adult daughter and her friends must have been having about her. The smile felt almost foreign. It had been a long time since she had smiled. In that moment, Maggie realized the impact her depression had been having on herself and her entire family. And she knew immediately that her daughter and her friends were right. Why hadn't hormonal changes occurred to her?

"Where did you get the pills?" she asked her daughter.

"From my girlfriend's mother, who went to see this person who's a nutritionist who helped someone else's mother who had a hard time too."

Maggie looked at her daughter in amazed gratitude.

When she came to see me the following day, Maggie related her story. We discussed how black cohosh had made such a difference to her emotional state. I explained to her how perimenopausal hormonal changes can affect mood and depression, and how her dramatic results indicated that she was on the right track.

After saliva tests, a few visits, and a few months on black cohosh and progesterone cream, Maggie's symptoms of depression, although much better, were still prevalent. At my suggestion, she consulted a physician, who agreed to put her on a low dose of natural hormone replacement therapy. Maggie also began using vitamin E as a complementary therapy, which in time enabled her to further reduce her dosage of natural hormones. Keeping the dosage down allowed the body to be more receptive to possible higher doses later if the depression got worse. This is a helpful option to reserve. Luckily the combination of natural hormones and vitamin E did the trick.

It is important not to underestimate the seriousness of some perimenopause symptoms. If ignored, some symptoms can give rise to a whole series of new symptoms. And the longer symptoms go untreated, the harder they can be to get rid of. Depression is a particularly debilitating condition, because it causes us to be vulnerable to many physical ailments and keeps us from fully participating in our lives.

Along Came Soy

How many foods can you name that contain soy? There are soy burgers, soy cereal, soy noodles, soy milk . . . even soy beer! Hundreds of soy products crowd our grocery store shelves while the media tells us that soy is a "miracle food," protecting us from every disease known to humankind. Because it is extremely high in phytoestrogens, soy has been recommended to ease perimenopause symptoms too.

But soy consumption is controversial. Some say that soy contains saponins, soyatoxin, phytates, protease inhibitors, and oxalate, which can impede the absorption of important vitamins and minerals. These may interfere with the thyroid (remember goitrogens), block the digestive enzymes we need for breaking down protein, and bind to minerals like magnesium, calcium, iron, and zinc, preventing their absorption. Even soy's isoflavones—phytoestrogens that are allegedly one of soy's most beneficial features when it comes to menopausal symptoms—actually disrupt hormonal function. In reality, the isoflavones in soy may contribute to infertility and breast cancer. On top of all this, it is estimated that almost 90 percent of soy originates from genetically modified plants. (I will discuss my grave concern with GMOs in more detail in a moment.)

We often see information about how healthy the Japanese are due to their high intake of soy. While it is true that statistics show fewer cases of breast cancer and heart disease in Japan, the numbers also reveal that the Japanese suffer from more esophageal, stomach, pancreatic, liver, and thyroid cancers. And, interestingly enough, the Japanese consume about ¼ cup of soy every day or two. In fact, they eat less soy than do many Americans! And much of what they eat has been fermented to remove the antinutrients. Too many questions about unfermented soy remain unanswered. I say it is time to say "So long, soy."

Keep in mind, however, that soy foods are divided into two basic categories: fermented and unfermented. Dating back to ancient times, fermentation is a process by which enzymes and microflora break down glucose molecules within food. Fermentation enhances the availability and absorption of protein. In addition, research shows that soy fermentation yields many other healthy nutrients, including calcium, copper, iron, magnesium, potassium, selenium, and zinc. And, there's more! Studies on a fermented soy beverage identified branched-chain fatty acids called small biosynthetic anticancer agents (SBAs) that are capable of inhibiting tumors. Scientific analysis indicates that these fatty acids act by inducing a programmed cell death—and can do so without any toxic effects. Combine that good news with the antioxidant properties of beta-glucans (powerful stimulators of the immune system that are present in fermented soy) and you'll see why fermentation is so beneficial.

Traditional fermented soy foods have been a staple of the Asian diet for nearly five millennia, and their medicinal and nutritional values are deeply rooted in traditional Chinese medicine. I continue to recommend moderate use of two primary fermented soy foods: tempeh and miso.

When it comes to unfermented soy, one of my concerns relates to the widely reported idea that it prevents breast cancer. It appears that soy isoflavones bind with human cell estrogen receptors and, by occupying space in these receptors, prevent cancer cells from finding a "home." Therefore, in some cases, soy is thought to protect against breast cancer. However, research has also shown that too much of the soy isoflavone genistein may lead to tumor development. Unfermented soy foods include fresh soybeans, whole dry soybeans, soy nuts, soy sprouts, whole-fat soy flour, tofu, soy milk, and soy milk products. In fact, most of the soy foods available in the United States are unfermented and overly processed!

As we have already discussed, the thyroid depends on iodine for proper functioning. Soy contains goitrogens that grab on to iodine, preventing it from being absorbed by the thyroid. For nearly seventy years the medical world has known about the negative impact that soy has on the thyroid. Yet some researchers remain conflicted about the validity of studies in this area, saying that the only people at risk for developing thyroid problems from eating soy are those people who suffer from borderline hypothyroidism already. My concern is that many perimenopausal women fall into this category.

The problems with soy extend to the younger generation as well. Owing to the estrogenic properties of soy, feeding infants an exclusive diet of soy formula is the same as giving them several birth control pills per day! Soy-fed youngsters may demonstrate an increased tendency toward zinc deficiency, premature sexual development, autoimmune thyroid disease, and diabetes. In several countries, including Switzerland, England, Australia, and New Zealand, the use of soy for babies and pregnant women is medically monitored.

Keep in mind that for years soy was not grown as an edible crop but rather as part of a plant-rotation process to add nitrogen to the soil. And today, more than half the soybeans grown in the United States are treated with pesticides that increase the amount of hormone-disruptive isoflavones. The bad news continues when you consider that

- as many as one in five people are allergic to soy;

- unfermented soy contains phytates, which bind to essential minerals, preventing absorption of those minerals (fermentation to produce products like tempeh and miso reduces the phytate content significantly);

- genistein can prevent normal brain function by inhibiting at least three metabolic pathways; and

- there are protease inhibitors in unfermented soy that may prevent pancreatic enzymes from digesting protein effectively (the fermentation process deactivates both trypsin inhibitors and hemagglutinin, while regular cooking does not).

We will no doubt continue to read conflicting reports about soy for some time to come, as researchers continue to try to resolve concerns about its safety. For now, if you are a fan of soy, stick with a serving or two per week of tempeh or miso or consider using Health From the Sun's fermented Soy Essentials supplement. But until additional long-term studies reveal the whole truth about soy, I prefer to recommend other natural options for dealing with the symptoms of perimenopause, including one of the most common complaints—hot flashes.

Is It Hot in Here?

The majority of women experience hot flashes during menopause, typically beginning about two years before the cessation of menses. Up to 50 percent of women continue having hot flashes for up to five years, while a few lucky ladies taper off after only one year. Some individuals experience hot flashes indefinitely. While studies are incomplete, it appears that African American women are more prone to hot flashes than women of Caucasian, Hispanic, or Asian descent.

So what does a hot flash feel like? While the experience can vary, it often begins as intense heat coupled with profuse sweating and ending with a cold, clammy sensation. A hot flash may disappear after thirty seconds or linger for five minutes. For postmenopausal women, hot flashes tend to be most disruptive at night. The changes in body temperature can cause frequent awakenings, leading to chronic fatigue, irritability, and mild depression.

What causes a hot flash? Hormonal changes in the body appear to create a vasomotor instability, causing a "misfire" in the body's temperature regulatory center. As a result, the heart speeds up and the blood vessels dilate, causing a flush of the chest, neck, and face. As the skin heats up, the rest of the body cools, causing a drop in core temperature. This explains why a woman may be burning up one moment and freezing the next.

For years, estrogen therapy seemed to be the only choice a woman had for getting some relief from hot flashes. Then, in a whirlwind marketing blitz, soy was touted as the natural way to soothe perimenopausal hormones. Now that love affair with soy is going a bit sour. Luckily, there are flavonoids superior to genistein for menopausal hot flashes, including hesperidin.

#10 PERI ZAPPER
Natural Estrogen Therapy

If the idea of horse estrogen and artificial progesterone (progestin) and the side effects—including a risk of breast cancer and unusual feelings in your body—doesn't sound appealing, you're in luck. Instead, opt for estriol (a natural hormone). After taking a saliva test to determine your hormone levels, you and your healthcare practitioner can determine the proper dosage for your body's individual needs.

Also consider taking phytoestrogens (plant estrogens), which can moderate your estrogen levels and ease your symptoms as you reach menopause.

So Long, Soy . . . Hello, Hesperidin

Hesperidin is a flavonoid, a colored substance found in many fruits that is essential for the absorption and processing of vitamin C. Bioflavonoids, such as hesperidin, are a class of water-soluble plant pigments. Hesperidin is vital because of its ability to increase the strength of the capillaries and to regulate their permeability. This helps reduce hot flashes by improving venous tone, restoring normal capillary permeability, and improving lymphatic drainage.

Like all flavonoids, hesperidin is not a true vitamin, per se, but was dubbed "vitamin P" by Nobel Prize–winner Dr. Albert Szent-Györgyi, the discoverer of vitamin C. It was in the course of isolating vitamin C that he came across bioflavonoids. He had a friend with bleeding gums and thought the condition might have something to do with a vitamin C deficiency. He gave the man some of his raw, impure vitamin C, and sure enough, the bleeding subsided.

However, when the condition recurred, Dr. Szent-Györgyi decided to try again. Using pure vitamin C this time, he expected to observe an even more dramatic result. No such luck. The man's gums went right on bleeding. The good doctor reexamined his earlier preparation and concluded that one of the "impure" bioflavonoids—and not the vitamin C—was treating the problem. As a result, flavonoids first came into use as protectors of capillaries, the tiniest blood vessels in the body.

Known as a citrus bioflavonoid, hesperidin is the predominant flavonoid in lemons and oranges, with the peel and membranous parts of these fruits having the highest concentrations. Therefore, orange juice containing pulp is richer in hesperidin than that without pulp. Sweet oranges and tangelos are the richest dietary sources of hesperidin. Like other bioflavonoids, hesperidin works best when given along with vitamin C.

Hesperidin deficiency has been linked with abnormal capillary leakiness as well as pain in the extremities causing muscle weakness and nocturnal leg cramps. Anticancer, antimutagenic, and immune-modulating effects have been seen with the use of hesperidin in numerous in vitro and animal studies. Among the cancers investigated in these studies are esophageal, colon, urinary, bladder, and skin. In one study that compared the cancer-inhibiting effects of a number of dietary flavonoids and bioflavonoids, hesperidin was found to be among the top-three most potent flavonoids.

Studies have shown that taking vitamin C and hesperidin over the course of the day helps relieve hot flashes. Although placebo effects are strong in women with hot flashes, other treatments used in trials failed to act as effectively as the hesperidin–vitamin C combination.

Hesperidin seems to work by improving venous tone, restoring normal capillary permeability, and improving lymphatic drainage. It also acts directly on the hypothalamus, helping it to regulate temperatures more easily. So to treat your hot flashes and restore your peaceful nights naturally—and safely—try hesperidin, 1,000 milligrams, coupled with 1,000 to 1,500 milligrams of vitamin C daily.

12.

Bioidentical Hormone Therapy

To Replace or Not to Replace

You read in the previous chapter what the whole-body effects are from too much estrogen, whether it be natural or not. Even on natural estrogen replacement, women still can have an increased risk for estrogen-triggered stroke and blood clots. And many of my ultrasensitive clients find symptoms of estrogen dominance, like tender breasts, headaches, and bloating, can even be triggered with mild phytoestrogens, touted in the literature as estrogen modulators. (Flaxseeds, we're looking at you.) The excess estrogen can also clog up the liver, keeping it from sufficiently detoxifying toxins, digesting nutrients, and producing the greatly important bile. This can leave you overweight, nutrient deficient, and on your way to hypothyroidism.

The estrogen replacement most doctors prescribe today for menopausal and perimenopausal women is a pill known generically as conjugated equine estrogens, a combination of estrogens derived from the urine of pregnant horses. Premarin is the best-known brand. Sure, horse urine may be "natural," but it is not natural to a woman's body. There are differences between horse estrogens and human estrogens. Equilin is the principle horse estrogen, and it is much stronger than any human estrogen. In fact, equilin packs a punch on the lining of the uterus as much as one thousand times stronger than human estrogen. No wonder Premarin increases the risk of endometrial cancer.

Provera (the brand name for medroxyprogesterone) is a steroidal progestin, the synthetic variant of progesterone found in Prempro. Since its invention in the 1950s, studies have shown that women who have taken it have experienced more heart attacks than those who haven't.

Estrogen:
A Pill in Pursuit of an Ill

In the 1950s, women who asked for relief from symptoms like hot flashes and vaginal dryness were told that these symptoms were all in their head. That all changed in the mid-1960s when the landmark book *Feminine Forever* by Robert A. Wilson, M.D., a New York gynecologist, introduced the theory of estrogen deficiency. No doubt influenced by his monetary ties to hormone makers, Wilson proclaimed that estrogen was the panacea that could cure any and every menopausal ill. He contended that without estrogen at menopause, women were destined to become sexless "caricatures of their former selves . . . the equivalent of eunuch[s]." Oh my! He brainwashed women with the enticing promise of youth, beauty, and sex, and women listened. They believed Wilson hook, line, and sinker despite the fact that he was criticized for making unsubstantiated claims.

Millions of menopausal and postmenopausal women started taking the "youth pill" as a magic bullet for their female issues. After Wilson's proclamation, other books and articles followed his lead, asserting the wonders of synthetic sex hormone supplementation—even suggesting it might prevent cancer.

Since their entrance into the marketplace in 1942 with Premarin, hormone manufacturers have created a major trend. They peddled their wares with a deluge of promotional books and films throughout the years, despite being backed by scanty science.

By the early 1970s, physicians were routinely dispensing both estrogen and tranquilizers. Thankfully, by the mid-1970s, research studies began to discredit the estrogen myth. In fact, in 1975, two studies appeared in the *New England Journal of Medicine* underscoring the connection between cancer in the uterine lining and estrogen replacement therapy. Then, in 1989, the *New England Journal of Medicine* presented evidence linking estrogen to breast cancer. When newer studies eventually showed that the addition of a synthetic form of progesterone known as progestin could protect women against uterine cancer, hormone therapy once again became the solution. Still and all, even with the documented dangers, by 1990, more than ten million women in the United States were on hormone replacement therapy.

Fast-forward to 2002. That was the year, as you know, that the Women's Health Initiative (WHI) was shut down three years early. As I have mentioned before, it was discovered that long-term use of HRT increased a woman's risk of stroke by 41 percent, heart attack by 29 percent, and breast cancer by 26 percent. Less than a year later, another WHI study of the effects of HRT on memory reported that older women on HRT had twice the risk of developing dementia. In Britain, at about the same time, the Million Women Study was halted when results indicated an increased risk of breast cancer and its severity among women taking hormone replacement therapy. Finally, in 2004, a Swedish study of menopausal breast cancer survivors on HRT was halted because of an unacceptably high risk of breast cancer recurrence.

The medicalization of menopause has not worked. We need, deserve, and are insisting on a way to regain our lives that is free from hot flashes, sexual decline, and insomnia, and that doesn't involve life-threatening side effects.

Natural, Bioidentical Hormones

A safer and somewhat more natural human hormone replacement can be found in urine excreted from the body of a young person for rejuvenation in an older person. In fact, doctors in Imperial China used such a remedy to halt symptoms of aging among members of the royal court. They evaporated urine taken from teenage girls and women in their early twenties. The crystalline residue of the urine was then combined with special herbs. The empress and women of the court were said to have experienced a regenerating effect on the skin, a boost in energy, and an improvement in libido. The same treatment was performed for the emperor and his royal court.

Although this may sound unappealing, this ancient "recycling" approach somewhat resembles today's estrogen replacement therapy with synthetic hormones distilled from horse urine. A much more compatible method would be using "bioidentical" hormones—hormones precisely identical to those found in the human body. These include estrogens, progesterone, and testosterone. Again, while no treatment—not even natural treatment—is perfectly safe, bioidentical hormones are much safer than horse urine estrogen or medroxyprogesterone. In fact, they may even decrease the risks of heart attacks, strokes, and cancer found to accompany synthetic HRT. Please note that even bioidentical estrogens, particularly in large quantities, have the potential to raise your risk of blood clots, which in turn can increase your likelihood of a stroke. Fortunately, these estrogen-related blood clots are easily preventable using omega-3 fatty acids and vitamin E.

Kate

At age forty-seven, Kate could live with waking up and feeling like a boiled lobster, throwing the blankets off, and waking up again a short while later, this time feeling like a frozen shrimp. It was when she started to put on weight for no discernible reason, on top of her constantly changing thermostat, that she decided something had to change. She always had led an active life and watched what she ate. In spite of carefully monitoring her portions now, and walking up every staircase in sight, there was no change for Kate on her bathroom scale.

She guessed that her problems had something to do with her time of life and came to see me because she was "not ready to give up yet." I told this tall, athletic woman that she need never give up at any time in her life—and least of all now. She and her husband had split up two years previously and she was now living alone, which she didn't like. I suspected that the stress of the breakup and the ongoing stress of her loneliness were associated with her hormonal problems.

Kate surprised me by refusing to have a saliva test to measure her hormone levels. I went along with this, in the hope that she would change her mind later when she began to feel that she was getting her weight problem under control. I didn't have to wait long. She had several hot flashes in a couple of days. Now she couldn't have a saliva test soon enough. The results surprised me. Her levels of progesterone and estrogen were both down. She was either much closer to menopause than I had imagined, although she was still having irregular light periods, or some other condition was causing the low hormone levels. I suggested that she try natural progesterone cream and take bioidentical estrogen, which her physician prescribed. She gradually built up her hormonal levels and achieved a balance. Her symptoms completely vanished. But she has not been able to reduce either the progesterone or estrogen dose without adverse effects. I would say that she is on the precipice of menopause, with the fact that she still has irregular periods. I expect that she will have a gentle, symptomless transition.

Having Your Hormone Levels Measured

The result of a hormone levels test lets you know immediately if something is seriously out of line. When you know what your hormone levels are, you can then seek treatment, if you need it, on an individualized basis. The test result gives you a baseline with which later test results can be compared, so you can monitor your hormone levels over time. When you have a hormone imbalance or low level and start treating it naturally, you should feel your symptoms ease and gradually fade away.

Delivery Systems

Today, bioidenticals come in many different shapes, sizes, and delivery systems. There are creams, pills, patches, lozenges (sublinguals), and pellets. The hormone pellet implantation has become increasingly popular. I warn you, I experienced this easily performed procedure in my integrative doctor's office and several months later had full-fledged periods once again with an increased uterine lining of nearly ten centimeters. I have heard similar horror stories from other clients of mine.

No matter what type of delivery system you choose, you will need to be closely monitored for natural hormone replacement—as closely as if you are taking synthetics. For most women, this is very costly, so proceed with caution.

You may not need bioidentical hormone replacement for very long. You may need to take it only as you move through the discomfort of hot flashes, depression, sleeplessness, and irritability. I routinely work with women who have been on bioidenticals for years, only to find that after a year or so they can't lose weight, they become sluggish, and their hormone levels shoot through the roof because they are *not* being monitored. They don't realize that as time goes on they need diminishing doses of the same bioidenticals. Be sure to work with your doctor to assess your ongoing hormonal replacement needs.

Still, if the natural bioidentical route is how you wish to navigate your perimenopausal journey, then pay attention to the safest estrogen of all: estriol.

Estriol

The body rapidly converts estradiol and estrone into estriol, perhaps because estriol has no carcinogenic tendencies. During pregnancy, estriol increases a thousand times or more to protect the fetus. Even after childbirth, estriol levels generally remain higher than before pregnancy. Evidence suggests that estriol offers many of the benefits of traditional estrogen-replacement therapies without significantly increasing the risk of breast or ovarian cancer when taken for more than ten years.

One notable study involved a participant group of fifteen thousand women, beginning during their pregnancies and following them beyond the birth of their children for thirty years. The researchers tracked all invasive breast cancer cases as well as deaths from breast cancer, and not surprisingly, their findings backed up the long-term benefits of estriol. The women who produced estriol in the top 25 percent during their pregnancies showed 58 percent less breast cancer during the study than the women in the lowest quarter production. Research conducted in a prospective style like this is considered more reliable than when information is reviewed after it has occurred, which makes this study particularly insightful.

Europeans use estriol extensively as part of hormone replacement therapy to treat the symptoms of the female hormonal transition. Estriol is a weak estrogen, so it requires larger amounts than estradiol when used in HRT. Symptom improvement seems to be dose dependent, meaning the amount of improvement directly relates to the size of the dose. But research indicates that the use of estriol even at high doses does not cause uterine cancer.

A large, long-term German study of estriol therapy for the treatment of menopausal symptoms found it was successful in 92 percent of all cases in eliminating or reducing hot flashes. Depression was improved by nearly 60 percent. Those pesky issues of forgetfulness, irritability, and brain fog also improved. Patients experienced a decrease in migraine headaches and remarkable improvement in vaginal dryness, plus a noticeable improvement in their skin quality.

Because it is important to consider how the amount of estriol compares with the amount of estradiol and estrone, you want to work with your doctor to determine the optimal levels of these three estrogen metabolites.

The Estrogen Window

Dr. Mache Seibel is a leading expert on women's wellness and menopause. Puzzled by what he considered to be conflicting information on HRT after concerns were raised in the Women's Health Initiative study, Seibel set out to resolve the dichotomy about the benefits and risks of estrogen. His research led him to identify what he calls the "estrogen window," a period of time during which using estrogen will maximize menopausal symptom relief and the associated risks will be minimized. "Estrogen isn't good or bad," claimed Dr. Seibel. "It's both and neither. It all depends on when it is taken."

The estrogen window is between five and ten years, starting when a woman begins menopause. Not only can women safely take estrogen during this window, according to Seibel, but also during this time the hormone provides a wide range of health benefits, including a lower risk of breast cancer, heart disease, and dementia. But women beginning estrogen after their estrogen window closes may increase their risk for breast cancer, heart disease, Alzheimer's disease, and osteoporosis.

Some Final Questions . . .
and Answers

Remember that information is power. This is especially true in the arena of health and nutrition. As women, it is vital that we all learn as much as possible about our bodies, the natural aging process, and the things we can do to be at our best—now and in the years to come.

It is impossible for you to take charge of your own health and your own perimenopause unless you educate yourself. And because the world of health care—and your own health status—changes continually, the opportunities for learning never stop! Here are a few common questions I hear from women as well as my responses:

I know I'm perimenopausal, but I'm only having occasional symptoms. What is my best course of action?

Your best bet is to meet any symptoms head-on by starting the Peri Prescription and incorporating one, or several, of the Peri Zappers listed in this book. You may want to begin with the mildest Zapper, flaxseeds and flaxseed oil. They often work wonders!

My doctor has been urging me to begin hormone replacement therapy. What should I do?

Be prepared to ask your healthcare provider some serious questions about HRT, including

- Why do you think I should take hormone therapy?

- What do you see as some of my alternatives to hormone therapy?

- Which hormone therapy do you recommend for me, and why?

- What are my current risks for heart disease, breast cancer, and osteoporosis? How will they be affected by hormone therapy?

Consider his or her answers carefully, along with what you've learned by reading *Before the Change*. The decision, as always, is up to you.

There is a strong history in my family of breast cancer. Is it safe for me to take HRT?

Because of the findings of the WHI study, most physicians no longer feel comfortable prescribing combination hormones to women who have a high risk for breast cancer. You should focus on the natural remedies discussed throughout *Before the Change*.

Since my mom died young from a heart attack, I was thinking that HRT might protect me from heart disease. What do you think?

I am sorry to say that the notion of combination therapy preventing heart disease is seriously outdated. Please do not use HRT to thwart heart disease. The new findings show that it doesn't work. In fact, hormone therapy increases the chance of a heart attack or stroke. And it increases the risk of breast cancer and blood clots.

Should I quit taking combination hormone therapy? I've been on it for three years for relief of menopause symptoms.

Because you have taken hormone therapy for five years or less, I suggest you consider tapering off the hormones and see how you feel. Keep in mind that the women in the WHI study were exposed to a variety of increased health risks within the first five years of beginning HRT.

What about me? I'm fifty-eight and have been taking combination therapy for nine years.

Chances are, you are past menopause by now, so try weaning yourself from the hormones. In doing so, you may "reawaken" hot flashes, but I've given you a number of natural options for dealing with those.

Should my mother keep taking hormone replacement therapy? She is seventy-two and has been on HRT for almost twenty years.

It is not wise to continue taking hormone therapy long term. In fact, the conclusion of another WHI study (published in the May 8, 2003, issue of the *New England Journal of Medicine*) was that combination hormone therapy had no meaningful effect on the quality of life of postmenopausal women. Boston's Brigham and Women's Hospital researchers Kathryn M. Rexrode, M.D., M.P.H., and JoAnn E. Manson, M.D., D.P.H., said that the WHI study "should challenge the widely held belief that HRT helps women remain more youthful, active, or vibrant." I suggest your mother taper off her HRT.

What's the best way to stop taking HRT?

The process of getting off your hormone therapy should be fairly slow, lasting several months. Doing so should ensure that you won't have a precipitous change in circulating estrogen levels, which can trigger hot flashes. I recommend using a natural progesterone cream, like ProgestaKey, available from Uni Key Health Systems (see Resources).

- MONTH 1: Begin your natural progesterone cream as directed. Take your synthetic estrogen pill every other day. If you use an estrogen patch, cut it in half. (Paper tape, available in any drugstore, is a great way to hold partial hormone patches in place.) If you take a separate synthetic progestin pill, such as Provera, stop taking it completely.

- MONTH 2: Continue using the natural progesterone cream as directed. Reduce your synthetic estrogen by taking one pill every third day or by using only one-quarter of a patch.

- MONTH 3: Carry on with the natural progesterone cream as directed. If you take estrogen pills, take one every fourth day. If you have been using the patch, cut it out completely.

- MONTH 4: You've done it! You are through with taking synthetic hormones, but you should continue your natural progesterone cream according to directions.

This gradual weaning-off process is the best way to prevent a recurrence of menopausal symptoms. However, if you do notice the return of hot flashes or vaginal dryness, try the Peri Zappers. They should do the trick!

13.

Clean Food and Pure Water

Cleaning Up the Contaminants in the Environment

I suspect that in some cases food and water contaminants are equally, if not more, responsible for symptoms of perimenopause than hormonal imbalance. But it would be futile to try to blame one contaminant or another, because symptoms so often are the result of a number of causes and can overlap. The hormone-disrupting environmental chemicals contained in impure food or water can make the body even more vulnerable to perimenopause symptoms. Viruses, bacteria, parasites, and chemical toxins enter the body through tainted food and water. Today, in an era of genetically modified food and rampant use of chemicals in the production of food and water, we also need to be wary of more complex environmental threats than simply exposure to germs from dirty vegetables.

It's downright scary. Many of us would cringe at the prospect of drinking jet fuel, yet depending upon your location, your water supply can be overflowing with invisible poisons like lead, chloramine (which has replaced chlorine as the major disinfectant in municipal water systems), pharmaceutical drugs, Teflon-like chemicals (PFOA), gasoline additives, and yes, even perchlorate, the chemical name for jet fuel.

These are but a few of the potentially lethal impurities found today in water.

All in all, more than two hundred industrial chemicals and neurotoxins have been identified in our environment. These caustic chemicals have been linked to decreased sperm count and intelligence as well as genital deformities, obesity, and cancer. Research strongly implies that each of us has at least some of these endocrine-disrupting chemicals in our bodies. In fact, in its 2008–2009 report called *Reducing Environmental Cancer Risk,* the President's Cancer Panel warned that babies now being born are "pre-polluted" due to their mothers' exposure to environmental toxins.

In light of the current information, we must come to the inevitable conclusion that we are all lab rats in a real-world, uncontrolled, largely unchecked experiment as a result of widespread use of chemicals. But cleaning up the chemicals that pollute our environment and have infiltrated our bodies is not so simple. Most industrial chemicals are not tested for safety before they are put on the market, leaving us in the dark on where to begin in terms of delineating their singular—not to mention combined—detrimental effects. Furthermore, the negative impacts of such chemicals aren't always immediately evident; the effects gestate slowly and invisibly until they mature into full-blown epidemics.

The phrase "clean food and pure water" has far wider implications today than it did a few decades ago, when taste and visual inspection were often enough to separate the good from the bad. Some of the most dangerous pollutants today are invisible and without taste. We need to know, as much as possible, where our food and water come from and how they have been treated.

All of this is why you must take your health back into your own hands. Make simple lifestyle changes to reduce your exposure to contaminants and become proactive in protecting your family.

Let's look at how to do just that. Not only will you avoid pollutants that harm your body and contribute to toxic overload, but also you will sidestep toxins that make your perimenopause symptoms worse.

How Pure Is Your Water?

Water is considered the universal solvent. It is vital at all stages of life, and, of course, perimenopause is no exception. Dehydration is known to cause fuzzy thinking, also a symptom of perimenopause. Water helps to lubricate dehydrated and parched tissues as well as aids the body to eliminate wastes. It keeps your skin glowing and your cells and systems working, and it delivers vitamins, minerals, and other nutrients to all your organs. For your glands to secrete hormones and for your liver to break down and excrete toxins, you need to drink plenty of pure water. How much? Most women should drink about three quarts a day, and it's always a good idea for anyone watching her weight to substitute a glass of water for a snack.

Make drinking plenty of clean water easy:

- Keep a glass bottle of pure water in your refrigerator at all times. (Stainless steel from China, by the way, can be contaminated with lead.)

- Drink a glass of water about fifteen minutes before eating to help quell your hunger pangs.

- Bring your own bottle of pure water when exercising or traveling.

- Drink pure water rather than soda or coffee, which can leach water from your tissues.

News of the water crisis experienced by residents of Flint, Michigan, has alarmed public health officials and consumers alike. And Flint is not the only municipality that needs to be concerned about water quality. Sadly, turning on a tap to fill a drinking glass involves an act of faith that in most places is not justified by the reality.

According to water purity expert Dr. Roy Speiser, "There are literally tens of thousands of miles of old and rotting water main pipes throughout the country—antiquated access ways that millions of Americans are blindly trusting to deliver reasonably safe, drinkable water. Some of these pipes are anywhere from seventy-five to over a hundred years old. Most are made of pure lead, concrete, or iron and as they erode, corrode, and disintegrate, residual toxins are leaching into the water that we drink, cook with, and bathe in."

The good news is that water is more easily purified than is food or air through point-of-use conditioning. Unsafe water from city pipes or country wells can be made fit for human consumption inside the home. But we need to remind ourselves constantly that water is not necessarily pure just because it comes from a modern municipal system or a rustic aquifer. All drinking water needs to be purified in the home.

Chlorination and Chloramination

For decades water treatment facilities have primarily relied on chlorine to keep us free from diseases such as typhoid, cholera, and dysentery. Many municipalities are partially adding chloramine to help reduce the levels of chlorine by-products and scum in pipes. At least we can be thankful that we don't get sick from tap water like people in many developing countries do.

Although we may be safe from things like typhoid and cholera, many studies have linked the drinking of chlorinated water to bladder and rectal cancers and also to some cases of stomach, pancreas, kidney, and brain cancers. According to the U.S. Council on Environmental Quality, people who drink chlorinated water have almost double the risk of developing cancer than people who do not drink chlorinated water.

While the intent of adding chloramine to water is to reduce the levels of chlorine by-products, chloramine by-products are also toxic and add more total disinfection by-product residuals. Chloramine is also known to be toxic to the kidneys.

You might question the wisdom of trading the risk of bacterial infection for the risk of bladder cancer. Many strongly oppose all chlorination of drinking water. Others suggest a change in its technology, including increased use of granular activated charcoal and bubbling of ozone gas.

Bottled Water

While there are various government regulations, namely through the Safe Drinking Water Act, to regulate tap water, no such oversight exists for bottled water. The FDA, not the stricter EPA, controls bottled water. It sets quality standards with allowable levels of certain contaminants. However, the FDA does not individually approve bottled water products or firms, does not have a set water-testing practice that these firms must use, and only inspects these firms if they have reason to. According to the FDA, bottled water companies are a low priority for inspection. Reading between the lines, you can quite obviously see that bottled water companies essentially have free license to conduct themselves as they wish. Unfortunately, as we know, we cannot always trust large companies to act ethically.

Standards are higher for imported than for domestic bottled waters. The permissible levels are a generous half-million bacteria per liter. Carbonated bottled water is likely to have a lower bacteria count than still water, because carbonation makes the water more acidic, which kills bacteria.

In addition to the water are the plastic bottles that contain it. These plastic vessels may contain bisphenol A (BPA) and phthalates, both of which have been publicly linked to lower sperm count and cancer. BPA is also a known xenoestrogen, with associations to learning and behavioral difficulties, obesity, diabetes, immune system interference, and, in girls, early puberty and problems with fertility.

There is one brand of bottled water, Penta, that I do recommend because it is natural and pure, free of chlorine, fluoride, bromate, arsenic, MTBE, and hundreds of other chemicals commonly found in some tap and bottled waters. Using a proprietary, patented process, Penta water is cleaned, processed, and stabilized for absolute safety without the use of chemicals or additives. Extensive research on the critical role of pure water is revealing new and exciting facts. In 1992, researchers discovered water-bearing protein channels in cell membranes called aquaporins, which manage the flow of pure water into the body. The research shows that the purest water—free of additives, chemicals, and even minerals—is what the aquaporins will first process to hydrate the body. This may point to why Penta water has superior hydration capability. It is available in many health food stores or from PentaWater.com.

Other bottled water brands I especially trust include Volvic, Acqua Panna, and Mountain Valley Spring, which is true springwater bottled in glass. All three waters include naturally occurring minerals.

Distilled Water

It might seem that distilled water should be the safest of all to drink. Just the opposite may be true. The process of distillation can vaporize and concentrate chloroform and some other dangerous compounds. Distilling also removes essential trace minerals from water, which anecdotal evidence suggests can cause calcium to leak from bones. For water to be pure, it must be double distilled. Few companies do this.

Hard Water

For water to taste and look good, and also to wash well and not clog pipes, its hardness should not exceed four grains per gallon. Hard—that is, highly mineralized—water was once believed to be good for our health. While it does contain essential trace minerals, its hardness is usually due chiefly to calcium carbonate, which our bodies need but cannot absorb in a desirable way from water. The calcium carbonate contributes to the blocking of our arteries and to arthritis, rheumatism, gout, and indigestion. It may also lead to bladder cancer or heart disease.

Treating Water at Home

My recommendation for water treatment is to use the CWR Crown AIO (All in One) Ultra-Ceramic Water Filter with Metalgon. This is the most effective water filter system available. The filter's method consists of three stages. In the first stage, tiny pores of ultrafine ceramic remove bacteria, parasites, rust, and dirt, all particles down to 0.5 microns in size. The second filter stage is composed of high-density matrix carbon, which reduces chlorine, pesticides, fluoride, herbicides, and other chemicals. In the third stage, a heavy-metal-removing compound, Metalgon, reduces fluoride, lead, and other heavy metals. Unlike some other filter systems, this system does not create an environment for bacterial growth inside itself, and it can be cleaned. A fluoride filter is also available.

Preliminary laboratory results indicate that Clean Water Revival's proprietary blended filter is effective in removing atrazine and glyphosate, two common chemicals used in agriculture (which we will discuss later). The filter is able to remove greater than 90 percent of atrazine from water, and it also tested very well in reducing glyphosate and other pesticides. The key is in providing enough layered filtration levels to be effective.

Comparing methods, one advantage of ceramic filtration over water distillation is time; it can take up to six hours to distill a gallon of water. The advantage of ceramic filtration over reverse osmosis systems is that it doesn't waste water, while reverse osmosis systems use three gallons to produce one gallon of drinkable water. (See Resources for more information about CWR's water filtering systems.)

Xenoestrogens

If you live or work in an urban or suburban environment, as most of us do, your body is subject to constant bombardment from petrochemical molecules. These molecules are in the air you breathe, the food you eat, the liquids you drink. They come from automobile exhaust, detergents, polychlorinated biphenyls (PCBs), and polycyclic aromatic hydrocarbons. As you know, their molecular structures are similar to those of estrogen, and they have the potential to occupy estrogen receptors in your cells. Breast cancer, enlarged ovaries, and premature cessation of ovulation are possible consequences.

Xenoestrogens in particular are a thousand times more potent than the body's naturally produced estrogen, meaning the liver has to work that much harder to process them. Even in the smallest doses, they can significantly interfere with the body's natural receptor sites, resulting in a slew of hormonally driven symptoms, such as depression, brain fog, headaches, and fat gain. Estrogen is a magnet for excess fat and water retention, making women with interference or unbalance in their estrogen levels vulnerable to weight gain. Add this to a congested, exhausted liver that cannot produce quality bile, because it is too busy dealing with all the extra estrogen, and you can see the impact xenoestrogens have on the body.

Xenoestrogens' effects do not stop at the liver and estrogen receptor sites. They may interfere with the actual manufacture of estrogen by the ovaries or adrenal glands, or decrease the rate of estrogen excretion from the body and cause a buildup of the hormone. Some dioxins mimic estrogen in the body, while other dioxins block estrogen's effects. Some xenoestrogens have widespread effects. For example, the fungicide pyrimidine carbinol inhibits the production of all sex hormones, not just estrogen. Other xenoestrogens have a much narrower focus: the fruit fungicide vinclozolin affects testosterone rather than estrogen.

I no longer need to tell you the dangers of unbalanced estrogen, so it should be obvious why you should avoid xenoestrogens at all costs.

In Search of Untainted Food

Three federal agencies—the Food and Drug Administration, the Environmental Protection Agency, and the Department of Agriculture—enforce a huge array of regulations to try to ensure that what we eat and drink does not harm us. As with all vast undertakings, there have been successes and failures, including, by these same agencies, oversights, overlaps, areas of controversy, conflicts, and bewildering behavior.

Food-Borne Illnesses: The Flu or Your Food?

Food-borne illnesses are the great pathological masqueraders. They often present themselves in our bodies as stomachaches, digestive problems, or even the flu, when, in reality, the culprit behind our discomfort is not a disease but last night's dinner.

Two recent food-borne illness outbreaks captured national attention. In 2015, Blue Bell Creameries faced a *Listeria* outbreak that resulted in three deaths and ten illnesses. The same year, Chipotle wrestled with a multistate *Escherichia coli* outbreak that sickened fifty-two people. According to the CDC, approximately forty-eight million people in the United States suffer the consequences of food-borne illnesses each year. Of these people, three thousand die. And these are only the confirmed cases from people who sought medical help.

Most bacteria, parasites, and viruses in food can be destroyed by adequate cooking (from 140 to 212°F). Proper cooking habits can virtually eliminate the risk of food-borne illness. However, various meats, dairy products, and vegetables have different temperatures at which they should be cooked to kill germs.

A Food Bath

To purify food, a special formula I use is the "chemist formula," created by my friend Larry Ward, a biochemist. The recipe makes one quart of solution that should be prepared fresh each day. In a quart of pure water, combine 18 drops of grapefruit seed extract with 4 ounces of 3 percent hydrogen peroxide and 1 teaspoon baking soda. Blend and soak all produce in the mixture (you can soak eggs as well) for at least fifteen minutes, then rinse well at least three times.

Perilous Pesticides

Experts continue to find evidence that genetically engineered and chemically sprayed crops threaten human health all the way down to the cellular and hormonal levels. Agrochemicals like pesticides, herbicides, and fungicides, even in the most minuscule amounts, can cause hormonal havoc to ensue.

Of these chemicals, glyphosate in Monsanto's Roundup herbicide sits at the top of the list. As I mentioned in chapter 3, glyphosate has been linked to cancer, a decrease in progesterone production, antibiotic resistance, and birth defects in rats, and it may have further endocrine-disrupting effects. It also, like gluten, does a dirty number on your microbiome, destroying beneficial, probiotic bacteria and encouraging overgrowth of bad, pathogenic bacteria. This can leave you with a dysfunctional gut, impaired immunity, and whole-body inflammation.

Billions of pounds of Roundup makes its ill-fated way onto the surfaces of crops every year, everywhere in the world.

Up next on the list is atrazine, an herbicide that is another one of the most commonly used agrochemicals. Dozens of peer-reviewed studies suggest that, like glyphosate, atrazine may disrupt hormonal function, but atrazine has a more pronounced impact on the reproductive system. It reduces estrogen levels and creates irregular menstruation. It may also harm fetuses and lower men's sperm quality. One study found that women who lived in areas with higher atrazine levels in the water had children with higher rates of some genital birth defects.

Other hormone-disrupting chemicals can cause the human body to respond inappropriately to stimuli, leading the body to trigger insulin production at times when it does not need it. The most common include pesticides found in foods; phthalates, commonly used in personal care products; flame-retardant chemicals, used in household goods, furniture, and mattresses, which may mimic thyroid hormones; and BPA, which mimics estrogen and is found in plastics and canned goods.

The Environmental Working Group publishes an annual list called the "Dirty Dozen," their Shopper's Guide to Pesticides in Produce. This list analyzes data from the Department of Agriculture and the Food and Drug Administration to determine which popular produce has the most pesticide residue. According to their list published in 2016, the top twelve fruits and vegetables with the most pesticide residue are the following:

Apples	Nectarines
Celery	Peaches
Cherries	Spinach
Cherry Tomatoes	Strawberries
Cucumbers	Sweet Bell Peppers
Grapes	Tomatoes

Veterinary Hormones and Antibiotics

As I pointed out in chapter 4, factory farmers gorge their animals with chemicals, such as hormones and antibiotics, in order to produce more product as well as protect against disease in unsanitary living conditions typical of industrial feedlots, CAFOs (concentrated animal feeding operations). Farmers and ranchers have six different FDA-approved hormones at their disposal, including estradiol, progesterone, testosterone, and bovine growth hormone (rBGH), a synthetic hormone said to increase the milk production of cows. A hormone in your hamburger or dairy product is a hormone in your body. In other words, these artificial hormone levels disrupt not only the livestock's internal environment but also the internal environment of whoever ingests their tampered flesh or milk. This can only add to a woman's estrogen dominance or excess. Notably, hormones are banned from poultry in the United States, but farmed fish are also given regular doses of antibiotics, and seafood harvested from polluted waters is exposed to heavy metals and chemicals, and may also be contaminated with hormone disruptors.

While there are no conclusive human studies, animal studies and correlational studies in people give reason to believe that antibiotics cause weight gain when consistently consumed at sub-therapeutic levels, as they are on feedlots. Furthermore, antibiotics without a doubt disrupt the microbiome, leading to digestive problems, widespread inflammation, and a slew of other physical and mental illnesses. Prolific antibiotic use also contributes to the development of antibiotic resistant "superbugs." As a matter of fact, in 2013 the Environmental Working Group estimated that at least one species of antibiotic-resistant bacteria, *Enterococcus*, had contaminated 87 percent of tested turkey, pork, beef, and chicken samples.

Go Organic

In a world where agribusiness seems to keep adding more and more chemicals to our food, organic food is trying to subtract.

In the United States, the Department of Agriculture sets the standard for what qualifies as organic for various products, including meat, produce, and cotton, emphasizing that "organic operations must demonstrate that they are protecting natural resources, conserving biodiversity, and using only approved substances." Certified organic products avoid synthetic fertilizers, chemical pesticides, and genetically modified organisms as well as work to maintain balance in the local ecosystem through their production practices.

Buying organic food can help assure that you are consuming food with minimal levels of added chemicals, allowing you to avoid hormone-disrupting toxins while maximizing nutritional benefit. So can eating in "farm to table" restaurants when you go out to eat.

To be sure your meat is free of drugs, hormones, and antibiotic-resistant bacteria, purchase organic meat, which by law cannot come from treated animals. Find a local farmer who raises pastured animals without chemicals. It is well worth any extra cost you may have to pay for meat from a healthy, clean animal.

In addition, the responsible farming necessary for organic produce lets you be sure you are getting the most nutrients out of your produce. Recall that factory farms, even if they produce healthy fruits and vegetables, have depleted their soil of nutrients through their farming practices. They rely narrowly on nitrogen, potassium, and phosphorous to enrich their soil and accelerate the growth of crops, instead of a full, diverse range of minerals. Fewer of these necessary minerals in the soil used to grow the kale in your favorite salad means fewer minerals in the kale itself, depriving you of the full potential nutritional benefit you could get from your healthy lunch. Organic growing practices work to maintain and replenish the variety of minerals in soil, creating more nutritionally rich vegetables and, therefore, more nutritionally rich people.

14.

Secret Cures for Perimenopause Problems

An Index of Lifesaving Tips

Before you pop a painkiller or turn to meds or over-the-counter drugs to treat the all-too-common ailments that intensify during perimenopause, I want to let you in on some effective alternative remedies. These are tried-and-true miracle workers from my work on the front lines of nutrition and are based on professional and personal experience. I do ask, however, that you follow instructions on the labels for most applications. Patience is the key; give the suggestions at least a week to kick in. (See the Resources section for where to order some of the products mentioned in this chapter.)

Allergies

To offset allergic responses to food or the environment, consider supplementation with up to 2,000 milligrams of pantothenic acid, which will replenish the adrenals.

Sometimes a mixture of quercetin and bromelain does the trick as well as Standard Process Antronex (a natural antihistamine) and MediHerb Albizia.

Gelatin is also astounding for people with allergies or sensitivities. It was one of the first foods ever used as a medicinal treatment in ancient China, supporting the mucosal membranes and providing a good source of amino acids.

All-Purpose

As a general remedy for all the miscellaneous trials and tribulations of perimenopause, you might try an essential oil remedy to help restore balance to your hormones:

- Massage marjoram, jasmine, or rose essential oil over your abdomen.

- Diffuse jasmine, geranium, or ylang-ylang.

- In a 5 milliliter bottle, blend 12 drops geranium, 6 drops ylang-ylang, and 4 drops clary sage, and fill the remainder with a carrier oil, such as fractionated coconut oil. Apply the mixture over the lower abdomen and lower back. For emotional support, rub it on the wrists and/or cup the hands together over the nose and mouth, and inhale.

Try Walnut Bach flower remedy or the Rescue Remedy combination to instill calmness and help you steady your emotions throughout perimenopause, or when you are going through something of high stress (for example, divorce or the death of a family member or friend).

You can also use your breakfast to fight perimenopause symptoms: oatmeal is a low-glycemic food that is an excellent source of fiber and good, protein-rich carbohydrates to support overall health. And use immune-enhancing nettles in soups or sauces.

The following herbs and plant foods are particularly rich in phytoestrogens, which we discussed in-depth in chapter 11 as helping to normalize estrogen levels:

Apples

Black cohosh

Celery

Chasteberry (*Vitex*)

Dates

Dong quai, or Chinese angelica (*Angelica sinensis*)

Elder flower

False unicorn root

Fennel

Fenugreek

Flaxseed

Honduran sarsaparilla

Kudzu root

Lady's slipper

Licorice root

Liferoot

Passionflower

Pomegranate

Sassafras

Soy, fermented and non-GMO

Thai vine

Avoid alcohol, sugar, caffeine, too much salt, and processed, fast-acting, or high-glycemic carbohydrates.

Anxiety

Vitamin B6 (pyridoxine) is very effective. It has been regarded over the years as "every woman's guardian angel" because of its role as a hormone regulator that stimulates dopamine, causing a calming effect on the body and helping you to handle the myriad stresses that can accompany perimenopause. Remember to take it with a B complex supplement, because the B vitamins assist one another in metabolism.

I like the activated pyridoxal-5-phosphate form the best for ultimate absorption and utilization.

You can also take a magnesium supplement (I like Uni Key Health Systems' Mag-Key, Dr. Sinatra's Magnesium Broad-Spectrum Complex, or a magnesium L-threonate) since a low level of this mineral can contribute to anxiety. Take 200 to 400 milligrams before bed.

As far as herbs go, black cohosh and kava can help ease anxiety. Discovered by Native Americans two hundred years ago, black cohosh has been widely used in Europe for more than forty years. Purchase a brand you trust. I like Remifemin, Metagenics, and Pure Encapsulations. Kava is also very relaxing.

For natural supplements, try the homeopathic remedy Nerve Tonic by Hyland's and StressCare by Himalaya.

Support your adrenals with this essential oil blend, so your body can have a more effective stress response and create less anxiety: In a 5 milliliter bottle, place 3 drops clove, 4 drops lemon, 3 drops frankincense, and 7 drops rosemary, and fill the remainder with a carrier oil, such as fractionated coconut oil. Apply the mixture over the lower abdomen and lower back. For emotional support, rub it on the wrists and/or cup the hands together over the nose and mouth, and inhale.

Breast Health

Natural compounds—such as DIM (diindolylmethane from cruciferous veggies), botanically grown medicinal mushrooms (like the maitake D-fraction extract from maitake mushrooms), Coenzyme Q10, and modified citrus pectin—contain immune-supporting ingredients that help prevent breast cancer and increase estrogen metabolism. Both iodine and iodide help to enhance the metabolism of estradiol and estrone into the "safe" estrogen estriol. I like iodine supplements such as Iodoral, SSKI, Iosol, or prolamine iodine.

Breast Tenderness

B complex vitamins can be helpful, as they break down excess estrogen, which can precipitate estrogen-dominant symptoms like breast tenderness. Sometimes iodine can also do the trick.

Try also the following herbal remedies:

Chasteberry decoction or tincture

Fennel seed and sage tea

Marshmallow

Brown Spots

There appear to be some potentially helpful new products on the market these days. Look for those with a daisy extract (like the Burt's Bees Brightening Eye Treatment) and/or licorice. Many of my clients have reported the fading of brown spots with BeauCle Corrective Creme, most likely due to a unique Australian anti-inflammatory extract and topical vitamin C.

Collagen

As we age, collagen starts to become depleted. Good sources of collagen include Great Lakes Gelatin and hydrolyzed collagen from pasture-raised cattle. Many women use a couple of tablespoons per day in a smoothie or in soups.

Topically, hyaluronic acid also helps to plump up skin and provides lubrication to the synovial fluid of joints. It's believed to hold a thousand times its weight in water.

Consider bone broth, which is teeming with collagen to soothe the gut and help replenish skin, hair, and nails. Use only organic brands, as non-organic can be high in lead and/or fluoride.

Reserveage offers a line of collagen-enhancing supplements that will come in handy for the perimenopausal body. Keratin, elastin, and collagen are featured in their special products.

Cramps

No, you are not suffering from a Midol deficiency, and forget that Advil or Motrin. Please, instead reach for magnesium and more B6, which have been shown to improve issues associated with perimenopause.

The following herbs are also an effective remedy for cramps. Some will work better for you than others because of biochemical differences between women. If some don't work, try others.

Bilberry extract (20 to 40 milligrams three times a day), or fresh berries

Black haw bark (cramp bark)

Chasteberry (*Vitex*)

Dong quai, or Chinese angelica (*Angelica sinensis*)

Ginger

Kava

Raspberry leaf tea

Red clover tea

Squaw vine, often taken with raspberry leaf tea

Strawberry leaf tea

Yarrow

You can also try the cell salt magnesium phosphate (6x), putting four pellets under your tongue every fifteen minutes until the cramping stops.

Black cohosh may help too.

Essential oils to try include black pepper, cypress, jasmine, and juniper berry. Rub a drop over your abdomen.

Cravings

Get the sugar out—a prevailing theme to overcome perimenopausal woes. Opt for more quality protein, fat, and compatible carbs (preferably grain-free).

Your sweet tooth may stem from an overgrowth of yeast. To kill the "fungus among us," consider oregano oil, SF-722 (from a castor oil extract), caprylic acid, or the homeopathic Y-C Cleanse (from Uni Key Health Systems).

I have found that taking 500 milligrams of the amino acid L-glutamine twice a day, between meals, takes care of cravings for sweets. Alternatives are:

200 to 600 micrograms of chromium per day

10 to 30 milligrams of manganese per day

3,000 milligrams of vitamin C per day

Depression

Eliminate all gluten and grains from your diet. Grains have been shown to disrupt microbiome function and subsequently cause inflammation throughout the body. Inflammation of the brain is a known contributor to depression. Add 1 to 2 tablespoons of flaxseed oil daily. Eat some protein and fat, and moderate your carbohydrates at every meal and every snack. When blood sugar levels are controlled, depression can also go away in some individuals.

Vitamin B12 is also a heavy-duty depression reliever. Make sure you select a methylated form of B12 for optimal utilization, and take it along with methylated folate to complement absorption and assimilation. It's always a good idea to check whether you have a genetic variation of the *MTHFR* gene, which can predispose you to mental illness.

The major success of Saint-John's-wort as a cure for depression has become widely recognized. This herb works better than tricyclic antidepressants—and without their side effects. Like Prozac, Saint-John's-wort is a serotonin-selective reuptake inhibitor. However, as with most antidepressants, you may have to take this herb for several weeks before its benefits are fully felt. The recommended dose is 300 milligrams three times a day of the standardized extract containing 0.3 percent hypericin. Half an ounce of dried herb per day can be taken as a tea or tincture. Saint-John's-wort is available in most health food stores. Photosensitivity is the most commonly reported side effect.

In the event that Saint-John's-wort is not right for you, try chasteberry.

Flaxseeds and black currant seed oil are helpful too, as is 500 milligrams of tyrosine three times daily. It's also worth checking for a hypothyroid condition.

Try melissa essential oil, also known as lemon balm, to alleviate depression. Diffuse or apply it topically to the back of your neck and over your heart.

Diabetes

Berberine is a standout to control runaway blood sugar levels in diabetics. It compares very favorably to the top diabetes drug metformin. Aim for 250 to 500 milligrams per meal.

Fatigue

Check for low thyroid and consider natural thyroid support (like Armour Thyroid or Nature-Throid).

Up your intake of iodine. We actually need two forms of iodine on a daily basis, which are iodine itself and potassium iodide. Your stomach mucosa and salivary glands soak up nearly as much of the element as the thyroid gland does. And iodine pumps are not only found in the thyroid gland and breasts; the ovaries, thymus gland, skin, choroid plexus in the brain (which makes cerebral spinal fluid), joints, arteries, and bones all have these pumps too.

For iodine supplementation, I personally recommend 1 to 3 drops of prolamine iodine per day or 1 to 4 drops of Iosol in 8 ounces of water. Since so many of my clients have Hashimoto's thyroiditis, I try to avoid any potassium-iodide-containing supplement, so I am cautious with Iodoral. Otherwise, for those with extremely high requirements and no sensitivities to iodine, one to four tablets daily of Iodoral works well.

To fight a loss of energy, try Ultra H-3, by Uni Key Health Systems, a remarkable natural remedy that also helps combat depression, arthritis, memory loss, insomnia, poor hearing and eyesight, graying hair, varicose veins, and heart disease—all without side effects so common with drugs.

Try out an adrenal support like Adrenal Formula from Uni Key Health Systems or some other similar formulation.

Dandelion, a liver detoxifier, helps in your body's processing of hormones, thereby relieving feelings of fatigue.

American and Siberian ginsengs have been used for centuries as tonics for fatigue.

BeeAlive's royal jelly line is a natural energy extender. BeeAlive's products are fresh and not freeze-dried, unlike other royal jelly products on the market.

Also known as *Eleutherococcus senticosus*, Siberian ginseng contains eleutherosides, which relieve fatigue, fight off infection, and promote endurance and resistance to stress. The recommended dosage is 100 to 200 milligrams per day.

Fibrocystic Breasts

First and foremost, reduce the caffeine in your life. Some have to go cold turkey and avoid all tea, chocolate, and caffeine-containing painkillers too. Many of these foods, like tea and chocolate, also contain theobromine, which is a well-recognized trigger of fibrocystic development.

Iodine can be a remarkable treatment for all types of fibrocystic breast lumps. Ask your physician to "paint" your cervix and vaginal area with Lugol's iodine solution, or take 6 to 8 drops of SSKI in a few ounces of water daily. This internal remedy may take up to six months to work, so patience is a key.

Natural progesterone acts to balance high estrogen levels that can cause fibrocysts in breast tissue.

Fuzzy Thinking

Even though your brain may be fuzzy, don't forget to get the sugar out of your diet! The Peri Prescription (with its healthful balance of blood-sugar-regulating protein, fats, and carbohydrates) is ideal for combating this complaint, as is natural progesterone. At the same time, it might be worthwhile having your thyroid gland checked out.

As a liver detoxifier, dandelion helps improve your body's metabolism of hormones, which does much to clear the mind.

In addition, try ginkgo biloba. Look for an extract that contains 24 to 27 percent ginkgo flavoglycosides and 6 percent triterpenes per dose. Then take 40 milligrams three times daily.

Ultra H-3 from Uni Key Health Systems is also effective for sharpening thought processes and providing mental energy. Take one to two tablets two times a day on an empty stomach.

Essential oils that improve focus include cedarwood, eucalyptus, frankincense, lavender, lemon, lime, marjoram, patchouli, peppermint, sandalwood, and vetiver.

Headaches

Evening primrose oil is an effective remedy for headaches. Headaches closely connected to the menstrual cycle and some migraines are best remedied with progesterone cream.

Once again, dandelion's role as a liver detoxifier that also improves hormone function can provide relief to bodily dysfunction, acting as a natural cure for headaches.

Copper imbalance can be the cause of migraine headaches and needs to be checked via a tissue mineral analysis or blood test. Request a test that will run a zinc, copper, ceruloplasmin panel for you. The key with copper excess or unbound copper is that it needs to be bound to ceruloplasmin in the liver, which acts like an escort. Ceruloplasmin can be strengthened with desiccated liver and/or vitamin A from cod liver oil.

Hot Flashes

Instead of sweating out a hot flash in the middle of the night, sweat it out in the gym. A Swedish study showed that women can lessen hot flashes by exercising vigorously for half an hour three times a week.

Another option is the herb maca. Maca works through the hypothalamus and pituitary to help ensure balanced and healthy hormone levels in the body. In addition, it is a powerful adaptogen, a substance that balances bodily functions. For example, an adaptogen will lower the blood pressure of a person with high blood pressure, and that same adaptogen will raise the blood pressure of another person who has low blood pressure. Try this balancing herb to relieve hot flashes.

The four best herbal remedies for hot flashes are dong quai (*Angelica sinensis*), licorice root, chasteberry (*Vitex*), and black cohosh. You might also try a decoction or tincture of chasteberry combined with sage.

The herb black cohosh is effective. Take between 4 and 8 milligrams daily.

An Ayurvedic remedy for hot flashes consists of *Aloe littoralis, Asparagus racemosus, Crocus sativus, Sida cordifolia,* and *Tinospora cordifolia.*

Dr. Tori Hudson's hot-flash formula consists of three parts sage, three parts peppermint, one to three parts motherwort, two parts gotu kola (*Centella asiatica*), two parts raspberry, one part thyme, and one-half part rosemary.

Dr. Hudson also recommends the following formula:

3 grams chasteberry

3 grams motherwort

3 grams unicorn root

3 grams wild yam

2 grams burdock

2 grams orange elixir

A daily dose of 400 to 800 international units of vitamin E is helpful. Vitamin E is really an E complex, which is why I like Jarrow's Famil-E. It contains all four members of the tocotrienols and tocopherols found in E.

Significant relief from hot flashes can be found by taking 300 milligrams a day of gamma oryzanol, extracted from rice bran oil.

Helpful essential oils include clary sage, eucalyptus, lemon, and peppermint.

Homeopathic remedies include Lachesis and Sepia.

Iodine is also a potent hot flash halter. Either Iosol, Prolamine Iodine, or Iodoral may do the trick.

Hysterectomy

For those who have had their uterus removed, hormone replacement therapy is essential for brain and bone health. I personally recommend bioidentical therapy, of course, but regardless of what you decide, do have your levels of progesterone, estrogen, and testosterone checked and monitored. Also pay attention to Peri Zapper #9, and support your liver and bile to clear any excess hormones from your system.

Insomnia

Low levels of magnesium in your body can cause you to wake up repeatedly during the night or to suffer from frequent sleeplessness. Many women have a magnesium-calcium imbalance during perimenopause. Taking a magnesium supplement may solve your sleep problems.

Mag-Key from Uni Key Health Systems is my all-around magnesium standby—as I helped to formulate it. Each capsule contains four of the most absorbable forms of magnesium, including magnesium glycinate to increase relaxation and mental acuity. Magnesium threonate, which targets the brain, is also helpful, and some individuals swear by Calm.

A GABA (gamma-aminobutyric acid) supplement promotes relaxation, antianxiety, and sleep. Doses ranging from 500 to 750 milligrams per day can work wonders to turn off nervousness and worry.

Kava has the ability to relax the body, making it a natural choice for the relief of stress, anxiety, and insomnia.

Valerian is well known for its sedative qualities and its ability to relax the central nervous system and smooth muscles. It has been used as a sleep aid for hundreds of years, especially when there is excitation or difficulty in falling to sleep due to nervousness. In a 1996 German study involving 121 patients, it took four weeks before a difference was noted, so you might have to take valerian for at least a month. The recommended dose is 600 milligrams daily, taken two hours before bedtime.

Essential oils that support sleep include lavender, vetiver, and Roman chamomile.

Keep in mind that intermittent awakenings can occur from surges in cortisol, created by malfunctioning adrenal glands or a parasite challenge. If stressed-out adrenals are the culprit, your insomnia may respond to adrenal support from Uni Key Health Systems' Adrenal Formula. If the problem is due to parasites, try cleansing your system using Uni Key Health Systems' Para-Key and Verma-Plus products. I have worked in the realm of intestinal parasites for nearly two decades and have noted that when an underlying parasite problem is addressed, sleep patterns also improve. It makes sense since many parasites, including amoeba, giardia, cryptosporidium, and worms, are nocturnal creatures.

Irritability

Magnesium, B complex, and evening primrose oil are almost guaranteed to help make you feel a lot less cranky.

Dandelion helps get your hormones working better by detoxifying your liver, which in turn makes you feel less irritable. Or try a decoction or tincture of chasteberry.

Natural progesterone can help; sometimes so can homeopathic Iodum or a natural source of iodine, like Iodoral or Iosol.

L-tryptophan can penetrate into the brain, where it functions as a serotonin precursor and works its magic before or one hour after meals. Take 1,500 milligrams twice daily with at least 25 milligrams of B6.

Dr. Jonathan Wright has recommended the amino acid glycine—the sweet-tasting amino—at 2,000 milligrams before bed.

Joint Pain

Glucosamine sulfate and chondroitin can help. The essential fatty acids from flaxseed oil, fish oil, omega-7 (anchovies and sea buckthorn), and evening primrose oil are effective. The mineral manganese can also be helpful for joint pain. I especially like Ligaplex I and II from Standard Process.

Hyaluronic acid, especially the liquid vegan Runovia, is supportive to cartilage as well as synovial fluid.

Leaky Gut

Bone broth does wonders to heal a leaky gut and soothe irritated mucosal membranes. Make it yourself or look online for organic beef, chicken, or fish bone broth.

Some individuals do well with added N-acetyl L-glutamine, as well as gamma oryzanol. Preservative-free aloe is also very soothing for irritated membranes (I recommend making your own with farm-fresh aloe leaves from Aloe King).

Mood Swings

Add protein and the right fats to carbohydrate-rich meals, and include the blood-sugar-regulating minerals chromium, magnesium, zinc, and manganese. Evening primrose oil is helpful too.

Support your adrenal glands with nutrients and supplements. Black currant seed oil, vitamin C, pantothenic acid, or licorice root can be a mood stabilizer.

The chasteberry decoction or tincture that eases irritability and other symptoms also helps with mood swings.

Wild orange essential oil eases anxiety and helps boost your energy. Cedarwood promotes a sense of belonging and grounding. Bergamot helps to increase confidence.

Osteopenia/Osteoporosis

My friend Dr. Janet Zand just reported an extraordinary testimonial that will be of interest to women of every age and stage of life. Here's what one of her fans told her of the power of prunes—a high source of bone-building boron: "I am now eighty-two and have had four bone density tests, which have told me I have the bones of a thirty-year-old. I'm told this is very unusual. One clinician told me that at the normal rate of bone loss, I will be a hundred and ten before I have osteopenia. Now I know why. For thirty-five years, I had a house with a plum tree and made prunes. I have continued daily use of four prunes for fifty years, thinking I was doing it for constipation. What a wonderful side effect to get these solid bones!"

PCOS (Polycystic Ovary Syndrome)

Try to lower testosterone by either progesterone supplementation or saw palmetto. Supporting the adrenals with adaptogens like ashwagandha and rhodiola (like Rosavin Plus from Ameriden) can also help.

Pelvic Floor Dysfunction (Pain with Intercourse, Urination, Sciatica)

A massage tool known as the Serenity TMT can help to stretch the pelvic floor muscle and help to release trigger points. This tool can aid in abating bladder, bowel, and sexual dysfunction symptoms while relieving pressure or pain related to the pelvic girdle, tailbone, or genitalia.

Periods—Heavy Bleeding

Clean up your diet by eliminating caffeine, alcohol, and spicy foods of all kinds. Stop smoking, also—the carbon monoxide and nicotine can prematurely halt egg production and damage the ovaries.

Natural progesterone often regulates heavy bleeding.

Massage rose or cypress essential oils over your abdomen. Or blend 6 drops Roman chamomile, 4 drops geranium, 3 drops lemon, and 2 drops cypress essential oils in a 15-milliliter bottle with a carrier oil, such as fractionated coconut oil.

The following herbal remedies are helpful:

Lady's mantle tea or tincture

Lady's mantle with an equal part shepherd's purse or yarrow

Cinnamon tea

Homeopathic Chamomilla or Actaea Racemosa (black cohosh)

Periods—Irregular

Try natural progesterone to balance your cycle.

Massage your abdomen with lavender or melissa essential oils. Also consider cypress, fennel, jasmine, juniper berry, lavender, peppermint, rose, rosemary, and/or thyme.

Homeopathic Graphites or Actaea Racemosa (black cohosh) are often recommended.

Periods—Painful

Massage your abdomen with marjoram essential oil. A warm compress placed on your abdomen can bring systemic relief. Also consider basil, cardamom, cinnamon, clary sage, coriander, cypress, dill, frankincense, ginger, jasmine, lemongrass, and/or peppermint.

Try dong quai (*Angelica sinensis*) tea or tincture, or lady's mantle with marigold flowers.

The cell salt magnesium phosphate (6x) can be helpful. As a natural muscle relaxant, 400 to 1,200 milligrams (taken to bowel tolerance) of magnesium aspartate daily is often helpful.

Homeopathic Actaea Racemosa (black cohosh) is often used.

Avoid alcohol and caffeine during the week before your period is due.

Sex Drive

Many decades ago British researchers discovered that *Panax* ginseng can treat atrophic vaginitis. This condition is typically caused by age-related atrophy resulting in thinner skin with no mucus production. *Panax* ginseng, taken over a period of three months, significantly thickened the mucosa lining, and women reported no discomfort during intercourse as well as the end of vaginal dryness. The dosage: 100 milligrams of a standardized *Panax* ginseng extract taken three times daily. Reduce the dosage after all symptoms have resolved.

Horny goat weed and maca are also revered herbal aphrodisiacs.

Surgery Precautions

All the natural remedies listed in this chapter are effective and safe for treatment of perimenopausal symptoms. However, I wanted to add a word of caution for those of you who require surgery for any reason. Please remember that prior to surgery, it's important to report your use of supplements to your doctor. Some supplements can inhibit blood clotting, affect blood pressure, influence cardiac function, cause sedation, or change electrolyte levels. Here are a few supplements that are known to affect the body during anesthesia:

FEVERFEW: This herb can be helpful for migraines and arthritis discomfort but can also increase bleeding, especially in people who already take anticlotting medications.

GARLIC: Despite all the marvelous benefits of garlic, you may want to avoid it prior to surgery. It, too, can increase bleeding time.

GINGER: While ginger may be effective in treating any postsurgical nausea, it has been known to affect bleeding time.

GINKGO BILOBA: Known for its power to keep our minds alert and our memories sharp, ginkgo can also lengthen bleeding time.

GINSENG: There is some evidence that ginseng may increase the heart rate and/or blood pressure during surgery.

GOLDENSEAL: While helpful as a laxative, goldenseal may worsen postsurgical swelling or increase blood pressure.

LICORICE: As a treatment for stomach ulcers, licorice can work well. Yet during surgery, it may cause high blood pressure, swelling, or electrolyte imbalance.

VALERIAN: This common sleep aid may increase the effects of certain seizure medications or prolong the effects of anesthesia.

Uterine Fibroids and Ovarian Cysts

SSKI to the rescue with 6 to 8 drops taken daily with 4 ounces of water. Results may take two to three months.

KBG (keishibukuryogan)—a traditional Japanese formula—is a potent healer. It is also known as "Gui formula" and is available through the Tahoma Clinic dispensary in Tukwila, Washington. This herbal blend is used in traditional Chinese medicine and is highly recommended by Dr. Jonathan Wright.

Vaginal Dryness

Frequently women going through perimenopause complain of an almost constant vaginal soreness or burning that makes sex extremely painful. Perhaps 80 percent of women suffer vaginal dryness at one time or another. *Consumer Reports* magazine found that more than half of its female readers used commercial lubricants to reduce unpleasant friction during lovemaking. A satisfactory vaginal lubricant—or personal moisturizer, as it is often called—is often harder to find than women expect because they contain petrolatum and other undesirable chemicals.

Oil-based lubricants were once thought to make women vulnerable to vaginal infection or irritation, but this has not proved to be the case in practice. In fact, I highly recommend MoisturePom, a natural personal lubricant that contains pomegranate extracts, olive oil, coconut oil, and coconut butter. Other suitable personal lubricants include Desert Harvest Aloe Glide and Aloe Life Personal Gel.

For very severe dryness, some women may need to get a prescription for estriol cream. Many women find it well worth the trouble to do so.

Carlson Labs' Key-E ointment or suppositories work well for many women and are found in most health-oriented stores and online.

The herbs black cohosh, dong quai, *Panax* ginseng, chasteberry, and he shou wu are beneficial for this complaint. So, too, are vitamin E, Remifemin (black cohosh), and homeopathic Sepia.

Avoid dehydrating substances (such as alcohol), antihistamines, and diuretics (including coffee).

Water Retention

Vitamin B6, taken with B complex, is a tried-and-true remedy for water retention. In terms of diet, watch salt intake and excess carbohydrates. Natural progesterone cream often acts as a natural diuretic.

Another effective remedy consists of shavegrass (horsetail), uva ursi, vitamin B6, and magnesium.

You can also try evening primrose oil or a decoction or tincture of chasteberry. Also try Roman chamomile essential oil.

Yeast Infection

Eat lots of onions, garlic, parsley, and living yogurt (dairy or coconut will do). Avoid sugar, cheese, white-flour products (such as bagels, breads, and pastries), fermented seasonings (such as vinegar and soy sauce), pickled foods, and foods containing yeast. These dietary recommendations often relieve allergies as well.

Drink lots of filtered water too.

The homeopathic yeast fighter Y-C Cleanse, by Uni Key Health Systems, is extremely effective.

Dr. Ohhira's Probiotics from Essential Formulas is an all-natural, superior probiotic developed to support digestive comfort and encourage your body's innate ability to grow its own friendly bacteria. Ingredients such as mountain springwater, fruits, and vegetables are fermented for three years, and the resulting nutrients from this fermentation process is called Postbiotics (a registered trademark of Essential Formulas).

Make a bath or douche of one part German chamomile vinegar to six parts warm water.

You can use goldenseal externally or as a douche, or myrrh essential oil as a douche.

For a watery but cloudy discharge, try homeopathic Pulsatilla. For a yellow, burning discharge, try homeopathic Sepia or Carbo Veg.

YeastGard vaginal suppository is also effective.

Avoid irritating soap and perfume, panty hose, and tight leggings or pants. Cut back on alcohol, caffeine, and fruit juices.

15.

The Peri Prescription

Your New Favorite Meals

Simply put, reprogramming your hormones through food can be quite delicious, and very doable! Just remember what you have read: hormones are the driving force behind many discomforting symptoms, like weight gain, irritability, acne, fatigue, depression, tissue dryness, and insomnia. Many times, if you do not deal with these SOS signals head-on, more severe imbalances can occur and morph into chronic conditions and more serious diseases. I'm talking about autoimmune disorders, diabetes, infertility, and breast cancer. Luckily, there are fast and simple dietary tweaks you can make to attain hormonal peace and enhance total well-being while improving how you feel and look. You've seen the science; now I will show you how to put it all together.

Basically, you will be eating the sexy, slimming fats (think mouthwatering coconut oil, butter, avocados, nuts) and quality protein (ideally organic and pasture raised) at each and every meal and snack. Both the fats and protein will definitely aid in maintaining level blood sugar and slowing the absorption of glucose into the system so you are satisfied throughout the day. You'll also be focusing on non-GMO whole foods, like leafy greens, colorful veggies, and grain-like seeds (amaranth, buckwheat, millet, and quinoa), with a moderate amount of low-sugar fruits, plus fabulous fiber (from chia, flax, and hemp seeds) and lots of flavorful spices and herbs that function as thermogenic and phytoestrogenic aids.

What you will be eliminating are the most common reactive grains (wheat, rice, and corn)—which can lead to inflammation or increased levels of heavy metals (arsenic, etc.) or cortisol—as well as refined sugar, caffeine, and alcohol. These substances can dramatically contribute to weakened adrenals as well as elevated blood sugar and more inflammation. I want you to avoid like the plague trans fats (margarine and partially hydrogenated soy oil) and commercially processed vegetable oils, often loaded with GMOs (canola, corn, cottonseed, and soy), because they can not only inhibit healthy liver function but also impede adrenal hormones. You'll also want to avoid as much as you can any foods that contain hormones or hormone-like ingredients, such as unfermented soy products and factory-farmed animal food products.

Smart Peri Sips

I have found that changing what you drink is a surprisingly beneficial first step toward better health and hormone recovery. So before you dive into the Peri Prescription particulars, let me say that when it comes to beverages, you will want to avoid most coffee (unless organic), black and green tea (with the exception of white tea), soda (both diet and regular), and alcohol for the most part.

Coffee, soda, and alcohol have devastating effects on calcium, magnesium, and the stress-fighting B vitamin levels in your body. Both cortisol-raising coffee and estrogen-raising alcohol can produce a dehydrating effect on tissues, while most types of tea are a surprisingly high source of fluoride, which can affect your thyroid, bones, and skin. If you must drink coffee, then mix in a tablespoon of coconut oil, which can inhibit strong cortisol spikes and provide a reliable energy source due to the metabolic impact of its medium-chain triglycerides.

I would mainly focus on filtered water between meals, as water is the best beverage of all. Water helps rid the body of waste, keeps tissues moist and lubricated, and can help burn calories. A mere 5 percent loss of body moisture causes skin shrinkage and muscle weakness—just what we don't need at this time of life. I suggest drinking purified or bottled water from a reliable source or a water filter for your home (see Resources).

Smart Peri Seasonings

I am not a believer in very low sodium diets—unless medically supervised and prescribed. I recommend using moderate amounts of Selina Naturally Celtic Sea Salt, Real Salt, or Himalayan salt for all your salt needs. Sodium is an important electrolyte often deficient in the perimenopausal woman.

Many natural spices act as hormone-balancing agents—like Ceylon cinnamon, which is helpful with insulin, and cardamom, a liver-loving spice that helps to modulate estrogen metabolism. Other phytoestrogenic herbs to use liberally include sage, thyme, fennel, and anise. Turmeric in curry is a natural anti-inflammatory, while mustard, cayenne, and ginger are thermogenic and stoke fat-burning fires.

Smart Peri Sweeteners

For special occasions, natural unprocessed honey, date sugar, maple sugar, and maple syrup are acceptable. I would much prefer these natural sweeteners that are a moderate source of minerals and antioxidants to artificial sweeteners or sugar alcohols, which can irritate the GI tract (like maltitol, sorbitol, and xylitol).

On a daily basis, if you need a little sweetener for your beverages or foods, stevia or monk fruit are great for perimenopausal health.

Just make sure that you don't let yourself get overly hungry between meals, which not only is bad for the adrenals but can wreak havoc on your pancreas as blood sugar levels plummet and shoot up too drastically. Make sure you pack healthy snacks with those sexy fats, fabulous fiber, slimming oils, and protein to take on the road.

The Peri Protocol

Now you're ready to put all the dietary components from *Before the Change* together in an easy-to-follow daily plan. This is a daily protocol that will ensure both happy hormones and optimum nutrition.

> 1 to 4 servings of sexy, slimming fats per meal
>
> 6 to 8 ounces or more of protein daily
>
> 5 or more vegetable servings daily
>
> 1 to 2 fruit servings daily
>
> 1 to 3 compatible carbohydrate servings daily
>
> 2 full-fat dairy servings daily (optional)

What follows are descriptions as well as lists of the foods you can enjoy and the portions I recommend. Mix and match to suit your own tastes—just make sure you get all the protocol requirements to fulfill your unique needs.

Sexy, Slimming Fats and Oils

As previously discussed, oils provide essential fatty acids (EFAs), which are of prime importance at perimenopause, because they nourish dry skin, hair, and mucous membranes as well as aid in natural hormone production. Oil also helps in the transport of calcium into soft tissues. The more of these fats you incorporate into your diet, the faster you will repair your hormones and even lose weight.

Just remember to add at least 100 milligrams of bile salts (or bile salt extract, as found in Uni Key Bile Builder) whenever you consume this premier food category in a main meal or in snacks to optimize digestion and absorption of fat-soluble vitamins and essential and healthy fatty acids.

Almost all of these glorious fats may be used in baking and cooking too—flaxseed and hemp oil should not be heated, but you can use camelina instead of flaxseed oil. These oils are included for their delicious nutty flavors and beneficial fatty acids, and many of them for their stability at high temperatures.

Each food source breaks down to equal about 1 tablespoon of oil, so you have the option to vary your beneficial fat intake from a variety of yummy sources:

Unrefined or cold/expeller-pressed avocado, camelina, coconut, flaxseed, hemp, macadamia nut, olive, rice bran, or sesame oil	1 tablespoon
Almond or other nut butter	1 tablespoon
Avocado	½ small
Butter or ghee, pasture-raised	1 tablespoon
Cacao chocolate (70 percent)	1 ounce
Coconut, shredded	2 tablespoons
Coconut cream	1 tablespoon
Coconut milk	3 ounces full-fat
Heavy cream, organic pasture-raised	1 tablespoon
Mayonnaise (made from avocado or olive oil)	1 tablespoon
Nut milk	3 ounces full-fat
Nuts (raw or home-toasted)	20 small
Seed milk	3 ounces full-fat
Seeds (raw or home-toasted)	1 tablespoon
Sesame seed butter	1 tablespoon
Sour cream, organic	2 tablespoons

Protein

Aim for one serving of protein per meal.

High-quality, clean protein is a good source of readily available iron, zinc, and vitamin B12, nutrients commonly deficient in a woman's diet, and important elements of the Peri Prescription. Omega-3-rich eggs are also a good source of minerals and antioxidants. They may be enjoyed daily unless you have an allergy or are suffering from gallbladder issues, in which case eggs are frequently contraindicated.

The following foods are excellent sources of protein provided they come from an organic source and/or are pasture-raised and unprocessed:

Beef, pasture-raised	4 ounces
Eggs, free-range or high omega-3	2 or 3
Fish (wild-caught salmon, sardines, or Safe Catch tuna)	4 ounces
Lamb, pasture-raised	4 ounces
Poultry	4 ounces
Rice, pea, or spirulina protein powder providing 20 grams of protein	1 scoop
Soy protein, selected fermented (tofu and tempeh)	4 ounces (2 or 3 times per week)

Vegetables

Try to eat five or more servings of vegetables per day.

Vegetables are very high in protective antioxidants and phytonutrients. Brightly colored orange and yellow vegetables—such as carrots, squash, sweet potatoes, and yams—are higher in cancer-preventing beta-carotene. Green foods like escarole, romaine, and arugula are rich in magnesium and vitamin A. Bok choy, broccoli, and kale are delicious sources of nondairy calcium. Each serving equals about ½ cup unless otherwise noted:

Artichoke

Bamboo shoots

Beans: green or yellow

Beets

Broccoli

Brussels sprouts

Cabbage

Carrots (1 medium)

Cauliflower

Celery

Chicory

Chilies: green or red

Chinese cabbage

Cucumbers

Eggplant

Endive

Escarole

Greens: arugula, beets, broccoli rabe, chard, collard, dandelion, kale, mâche, mustard, radicchio, spinach, or turnip

Jerusalem artichoke (sunchoke)

Jicama

Mushrooms

Okra

Onions

Peppers: green or red

Radishes: daikon or red

Sauerkraut

Seaweed: kelp or nori

Snow peas

Sprouts: adzuki, alfalfa, clover, mung bean, or radish

Squash: chayote, spaghetti, or summer

Tomatoes

Tomato juice

Vegetable juice cocktail

Water chestnuts (4)

Watercress

Zucchini

Fruits

Aim for 2 or 3 servings per day from the fruit group.

Many women eat too much fruit in the mistaken belief that because fruit is natural it can be eaten without limits. Too much fruit, no matter what the source, can upset the delicate calcium balance in the system and increase triglyceride levels. Fruit is also a hidden source of fructose—one of the highly suspected underlying causes of non-alcoholic fatty liver, which is on the rise, and elevated triglycerides. High-fructose fruits include many dried fruits, so they should be enjoyed in moderation—for special occasions (two dates, figs, prunes, or apricots, or 2 tablespoons raisins). If yeast problems are a concern, temporarily avoid all fruits for at least two weeks.

Apple	1 small
Banana	½ small
Berries: blackberries, blueberries, boysenberries, loganberries, or raspberries	½ cup
Cantaloupe	¼ medium
Cherries	10 large

Grapefruit	½ small
Kiwi	1 medium
Mango	½ cup
Nectarine	1 small
Orange	1 small
Orange juice (unsweetened)	½ cup
Papaya	½ cup
Peach	1 medium
Pear	1 small
Persimmon	1 medium
Pineapple	½ cup
Plums	2 medium
Pomegranate	1 small
Tangerine	1 large
Watermelon	1 cup

Dairy Products

I recommend up to two portions of dairy food per day (optional).

If you are sensitive to dairy because of lactose or casein intolerance, then ditch it entirely and opt for coconut substitutes. If you suffer from adult acne, it's best to avoid this food group, because the hormones in even organic and pasture-raised dairy can wreak havoc on the skin.

Cottage cheese (full-fat)	½ cup
Feta cheese (imported)	½ cup
Greek yogurt (full-fat)	1 cup
Hard cheese (aged at least 6 months)	1 ounce

| Kefir | 1 cup |
| Ricotta cheese (full-fat) | ½ cup |

Compatible Carbs

Aim for 1 to 3 servings per day from this family of foods.

Starchy veggies, like beets, pumpkins, squash, and sweet potatoes, should be your hormonal mainstay. These veggies provide high amounts of antioxidants and natural sweetness. Fiber-rich seed grains, such as amaranth, buckwheat, millet, oats, and quinoa, are recommended for their high magnesium content and should be eaten instead of the more highly reactive grains, like wheat, rice, and corn.

Legumes are good non-animal protein and iron sources. Dried beans, lentils, and peas are tops in high fiber, with from 4 to 8 grams per serving.

Amaranth and quinoa are two very healthy grain-like seeds. These grains have a buttery, rich flavor. Amaranth, a tiny grain seed that is a fairly new addition to store shelves, was widely used by the Aztecs in Mexico hundreds of years ago and was revered as a magical, mystical grain. It is one of the highest protein grains, at 16 percent. A ½ cup cooked serving also has as much calcium as an 8-ounce glass of milk. Amaranth is a good source of lysine and methionine, essential amino acids lacking in almost all other grains. This unusual grain can be used alone as a cereal or added to the batter of breads and baked goods. In protein value, quinoa is as high as or higher than amaranth. Known as the "mother grain" of the Incas, quinoa is low in gluten but is an abundant source of the amino acids methionine and cysteine as well as lysine. Both of these grains are used as cereals and flour and are available without pesticides and sprays.

Starchy Vegetables

Beets	½ cup
Chestnuts	4 large or 6 small
Corn (cooked)	⅓ cup

Corn (on the cob)	1 (4 inches long)
Parsnips	1 small
Peas (fresh)	¼ cup
Potatoes: sweet or white	1 small
Potatoes: sweet or white (mashed)	½ cup
Pumpkin	⅓ cup
Rutabaga	1 small
Squash (winter types)	½ cup
Succotash	½ cup
Turnips	1 small
Yam	1 small

Flours

Almond	3 tablespoons
Arrowroot	2 tablespoons
Coconut	3 tablespoons
Kuzu (root starch)	2 tablespoons
Almond or cassava and coconut tortilla (Siete brand)	1 regular

Legumes

Beans: black, garbanzo (chickpeas), kidney, lima, navy, pinto, (cooked)	½ cup
Lentils (cooked)	½ cup
Peas (cooked)	½ cup

Nutritional Supplementation

As a nutritionist, I believe—and I know my clients do too—that food is our best source of vitamins, minerals, enzymes, and amino acids for health. But because of hectic schedules, we can't always eat the way we know we should. To make matters worse, topsoil is now depleted of certain trace minerals that are important for health, due largely to factory farming—minerals such as zinc, chromium, selenium, and magnesium. The stress of modern-day life, environmental pollution, and radiation all take their nutrient tolls on the twentieth-century body. Supplemental vitamins and minerals have become a necessity, not a luxury. It is no wonder that more than a hundred million Americans are supplementing their diets.

In light of these situational constraints and the major glandular shifts occurring during the prime of our lives, I recommend for my clients a special comprehensive regimen to help meet their unique nutritional needs. Full disclosure: I am a spokesperson for Uni Key Health Systems and have helped to formulate many of their products, so I am most familiar with the efficacy of their formulations. You can choose to use their name-brand products or look online and find similar formulations at your local health food store. I have also included other name-brand formulations that I especially like.

HCl digestive aid (hydrochloric acid and pepsin)	1 or 2 capsules, three times a day
Jarrow Famil-E (vitamin E support)	400 IU, three times a day
LifeExtension Berberine	250 milligrams, three times a day with meals
Natural progesterone body cream	¼ to ½ teaspoon, two times a day
Uni Key Adrenal Formula	2 capsules, three times a day
Uni Key Bile Builder	1 or 2 capsules, with each meal

| Uni Key Female Multiple (copper-free) | 2 capsules, three times a day |
| Uni Key Mag-Key (magnesium support) | 5 milligrams per pound of body weight per day |

For my diabetic clients and those who crave sugar, I add 200 micrograms chromium, two times per day. These supplements can be ordered directly from Uni Key Health Systems, my fulfillment center for all products, tests, and services, at 800-888-4353. Please remember that individual requirements may vary.

Mindful Medicine

Prescription drugs and over-the-counter medications can interfere with the digestion and absorption of key nutrients. For example, antibiotics and antacids affect calcium utilization. Diuretics eliminate potassium, zinc, and magnesium. Aspirin interferes with vitamin C and iron absorption, and can also magnify the effects of other medications, such as blood thinners. If you are taking prescription drugs, try to eat foods high in vitamins that the medication depletes, or consider vitamin supplementation.

It is helpful to know about drug interactions so as to avoid reactions. Make sure that your primary physician is aware of every single prescription drug and over-the-counter medication you are taking. (In this age of medical specialists, it is common for people to see different physicians for different health concerns, getting medications from each doctor, none of whom may be aware of the others' prescriptions.) Some drugs can cancel out the effect of others or magnify their potency. You should know all potential side effects, whether your medicine should be taken with meals or without food, and the length of time you should be on it.

Cooking Utensils

It is best to avoid all aluminum-containing pots, pans, and foil, because aluminum hampers the body's utilization of calcium and phosphorus. High-quality stainless steel, cast iron, enamel-covered iron, Corning-Ware, Pyrex, and other heat-resistant glass are preferable.

The real danger of aluminum comes from the aluminum hydroxides in many antacids, baking powder, and baking soda, and in the fluoride that is in aluminum foil. If you are going to freeze or refrigerate in aluminum foil, it is best to first wrap with waxed paper and then use the aluminum, so that none will leach into your food.

Putting It All Together

Now you're prepared to enter into this new phase of your life and manage menopause the *Before the Change* way. Your transition to a diet low in processed foods and rich in nutrients, and your commitment to a consistent exercise regimen, will help ease you naturally into midlife.

Sample Menu

The sample one-week menu and recipes are based on the Peri Protocol. They are designed to avoid dietary culprits like altered fats, gluten-rich grains, sugars, and GMO foods. By avoiding these common pitfalls, hormones will be reprogrammed, digestion will be enhanced, and well-being will be boosted all around. Please note that menu items with page numbers appear in the recipe section that follows.

Day 1

BREAKFAST: Banana Float Smoothie (page 246)

LUNCH: 4 ounces baked salmon on mixed lettuces with 1 to 2 tablespoons Pretty in Pesto Dressing (page 246)

DINNER: 2 cups cooked spaghetti squash topped with 4 ounces ground beef, cooked, topped with 1 cup no-sugar-added tomato sauce mixed with garlic and Italian herbs, served with a side of ½ cup cooked millet

SNACK: 1 medium Granny Smith apple, sliced, rolled in 1 tablespoon flaxseeds

Day 2

BREAKFAST: Parfait of 8 ounces Greek yogurt with ½ cup mixed berries plus 1 tablespoon flaxseed oil and 1 tablespoon hemp seeds

LUNCH: 4-ounce turkey burger on portobello mushroom caps with sliced cucumbers and red peppers, topped with 1 tablespoon olive oil and dill

DINNER: 4 ounces lamb chops broiled with rosemary, and ½ cup asparagus drizzled with 1 tablespoon sesame oil, plus ½ cup peas with mint

SNACK: ½ grapefruit topped with 1 tablespoon sunflower seeds

Day 3

BREAKFAST: 2 eggs fried in avocado oil, with ½ cup steamed spinach and garlic with 1 tablespoon flaxseeds

LUNCH: Salad with 4 ounces shrimp plus mung bean sprouts and shredded cabbage mixed with 1 tablespoon sesame seed oil and 1 teaspoon sesame seeds

DINNER: 4 ounces chicken broiled with rosemary and garlic, with leeks and zucchini sautéed in 1 tablespoon olive oil, served over ½ cup cooked buckwheat grouts

SNACK: ½ cantaloupe with 2 tablespoons cashew butter

Day 4

BREAKFAST: ½ grapefruit with 4 ounces scrambled tofu with 2 slices turkey bacon

LUNCH: 4 ounces ground beef in 1 almond or cassava and coconut tortilla topped with 1 tablespoon sour cream and shredded lettuces

DINNER: 4 ounces chicken cooked in a slow cooker with 4 ounces sauerkraut, string beans, and yellow squash with ½ cup cooked and cooled quinoa with parsley and onions drizzled with 1 tablespoon flaxseed oil

SNACK: 2 jicama sticks topped with 2 tablespoons pumpkin-seed butter

Day 5

BREAKFAST: Chocolate Crème Smoothie (see Variation, page 246)

LUNCH: 4 ounces crab shredded with ½ avocado and juice of ½ lemon, plus onion and celery salad with 1 tablespoon flaxseed oil

DINNER: Stir-fry with 4 ounces tofu or tempeh with ½ cup butternut squash, bok choy, and fennel with 1 tablespoon toasted sesame seed oil

SNACK: Handful of pecans and 1 tangerine

Day 6

BREAKFAST: ½ cup cottage cheese and ½ cup pineapple with 1 tablespoon flaxseeds

LUNCH: 4 ounces tuna fish mixed with 1 hard-boiled egg, 1 tablespoon curry powder, and ½ cup chopped celery on top of ½ avocado

DINNER: 4 ounces flank steak marinated in lime juice and olive oil, with sweet potato (1 small) and cauliflower "rice"

SNACK: 1 cup yogurt with ½ cup mango and 2 tablespoons sliced toasted almonds

Day 7

BREAKFAST: Almond or cassava and coconut tortilla steamed and topped with 1 ounce swiss cheese, melted

LUNCH: 1 cup Greek Lentil Soup (page 247) with leafy green salad and 1 tablespoon flaxseed oil

DINNER: Chicken fajitas with 4 ounces chicken strips wrapped in romaine lettuce leaves with salsa, and steamed broccoli and yellow squash topped with pine nuts

SNACK: 10 frozen cherries, or Silky Chocolate Avocado Pudding (page 248)

Recipes

Banana Float Smoothie

Serves 1

½ ripe banana
1 scoop vanilla protein powder (Uni Key Body Protein or
   Whey Protein, or other)
8 ounces almond milk
1 tablespoon almond butter
1 tablespoon flaxseed oil
4 ice cubes

Place all ingredients in a blender and blend until smooth.

VARIATION: For the Chocolate Crème Smoothie, use chocolate whey protein in place of the vanilla, and use coconut milk to replace the almond milk.

Pretty in Pesto Dressing

Makes about 1 cup

2 cups chopped parsley
¾ cup pine nuts, toasted
4 garlic cloves, chopped
½ cup extra-virgin olive oil
½ cup chopped beets
½ teaspoon sea salt
2 tablespoons fresh lemon juice

Combine the parsley, pine nuts, garlic, olive oil, and beets in a blender or food processor.

Just before serving, stir in the salt and lemon.

Greek Lentil Soup

Serves 4

1 cup lentils, washed and soaked in 4 cups water overnight
3 cups water
1 tablespoon extra-virgin olive oil
1 tablespoon fresh lemon juice
1 onion, chopped
1 carrot, chopped
½ cup chopped green pepper
1 celery stalk with leaves, chopped
1 garlic clove, minced
2 tablespoons chopped fresh parsley
½ bay leaf
¾ teaspoon salt (optional)
½ teaspoon mustard seed
½ teaspoon ground cumin
2 tablespoons finely chopped green onions, for garnish

Drain the soaked lentils, and place them in the 3 cups water in a covered pot.

Bring the water to a boil and simmer.

Add the olive oil and lemon juice.

Cook for 30 minutes until the lentils are tender.

Add the onion, carrot, green pepper, celery, garlic, parsley, bay leaf, salt (if using), mustard seed, and cumin.

Simmer, covered, for an additional 20 to 30 minutes, until the vegetables are tender.

Serve topped with the green onions for garnish, if using.

Silky Chocolate Avocado Pudding

Serves 1 or 2

2 ripe avocados, skinned
⅛ cup full-fat coconut milk
2 tablespoons unsweetened cocoa powder
1 teaspoon NutraMedix Stevia Liquid
1 ounce dark chocolate (70 percent cacao), melted
1 teaspoon vanilla extract
¼ teaspoon salt

Place all the ingredients in a blender and blend until smooth and silky.

Pour the mixture into a sealable container, seal, and let the pudding set in the refrigerator for at least 12 hours before serving.

Resources

Connect with Ann Louise

Please visit me online at www.annlouise.com and on Facebook at facebook.com/annlouisegittleman. Visitors to my website and subscribers to my email list never miss my latest blogs and are the first to know about news and upcoming events. Plus, you can stay up-to-date with my latest webinars, summits, podcasts, and television appearances.

Uni Key Health Systems

Uni Key Health Systems has been my go-to distributor for many supplements and test kits for more than twenty-five years. It was founded in 1992 by James Templeton, a cancer survivor who used alternative medicine to heal himself. His mission is now to help others find the root causes of disease and heal themselves with drug-free methods. Uni Key Health proudly provides high-quality nutritional supplements, vitamins, and health information for diet/detox, weight loss, cleansing, antiaging, energy, hormonal balance, and skin care. Full disclosure: I have been a spokesperson and formulator for Uni Key Health Systems for more than twenty years.

> 181 West Commerce Drive
> Hayden Lake, ID 83835
> 800-888-4353
> www.unikeyhealth.com

Peri-appropriate supplements available from Uni Key include:

Adrenal Formula

Bile Builder

Carlson Fish Oil Softgels

CLA-1000

Dandelion Root Tea

Fat Flush Body Protein (non-GMO from vegan rice and pea)

Fat Flush Whey Protein (from hormone-free non-mutated A2 milk protein)

Female Multiple

GLA-90 (from black currant seed oil)

Liver-Lovin Formula

Mag-Key

Omega Nutrition Cold Milled Flaxseeds

Omega Nutrition Organic Flax Oil

ProgestaKey

Also available from Uni Key:

EARTHING PRODUCTS: Reconnect to the earth's natural healing electrons with products designed to ground yourself for better sleep, increased endurance, enhanced energy, and overall balance.

SALIVARY HORMONE TEST: Unlike blood tests, which do not measure bioavailable hormone activity, saliva testing is considered to be the most accurate measure of free, bioavailable hormonal activity. This personal hormone evaluation can be used to profile up to six hormones: estradiol, estriol, progesterone, testosterone, DHEA, and cortisol. Your personal results and a personal letter of recommendation from my office are mailed directly to your home.

TISSUE MINERAL ANALYSIS: This test uses a small sample of hair cut from the back of your head. This analysis includes a full report, up to twenty pages, which graphically shows the levels of thirty-two major minerals and six toxic metals in the body. Each mineral is fully evaluated in terms of its relationship with other minerals, which is a key to glandular function and metabolism rate. This report provides information on the effect of vitamin deficiency and excesses. There is also a complete discussion regarding environmental influences and disease tendencies based upon mineral levels and ratios. A list of recommended food choices and supplements, based upon the individual findings, is included at the end of the report.

WATER FILTRATION: Purify your water to protect against harmful chemicals and toxins, parasites like giardia and amoeba, chloromines, and heavy metals. A water quality consultation is available with a filtration expert free of charge.

Other Products

BACH FLOWER REMEDIES: For the renowned remedies developed by English immunologist Dr. Edward Bach in the 1930s. The most renowned formula, Rescue Remedy, is a five-flower extract combo used to help alleviate trauma, whether emotional, physical, or psychological.
800-214-2850
www.bachflower.com

BARLEAN'S: For non-GMO omega-rich oils, including Barlean's, and for Heart Remedy Omega-7 Omega Swirl, which I've found to be the most tasty (and least fishy) anchovy oil on the market.
800-445-3529
www.barleans.com

ESSENTIAL FORMULAS: For Dr. Ohhira's Probiotics and Reg'Activ by Essential Formulas, the liver-targeted probiotic formula containing the revolutionary *Lactobacillus fermentum* ME-3 strain.
972-255-3918
www.essentialformulas.com

MAINE SEAWEED: For high-quality sea vegetables, located in the northeastern United States.
207-546-2875
https://theseaweedman.com

SELINA SEA SALT: For the highest-quality Celtic sea salts. I especially love their Makai Pure Deep Sea Salt with the highest potassium level of any comparable sea salt on the market.
800-867-7258
www.selinanaturally.com

Women's Health

CLEAR PASSAGE—PHYSICAL THERAPY & PHYSIOTHERAPY: Over the years, the Clear Passage group has developed, tested, and published results on protocols that are effective in treating a wide variety of adhesion-related conditions, including female infertility, endometriosis, hormonal conditions, postsurgical pain, and bowel obstructions.
866-222-9437 or 352-336-1433
www.clearpassage.com

HEALTHYWOMEN: HW is a leading independent health information source for women. Their core mission is to educate, inform, and empower women to make smart health choices for themselves and their families.
877-986-9472
www.healthywomen.org

PELVIC FLOOR THERAPY AND PRACTITIONERS

Canada
PELVIC HEALTH SOLUTIONS
online directory
http://pelvichealthsolutions.ca/find-a-health-care
-professional

USA

HERMAN & WALLACE PELVIC REHABILITATION INSTITUTE
online directory
https://hermanwallace.com/practitioner-directory

SECTION ON WOMEN'S HEALTH
online directory
www.womenshealthapta.org/pt-locator

RECOMMENDED PRIVATE PRACTITIONERS IN THE UNITED STATES

JESSICA DRUMMOND, M.P.T., C.C.N., C.H.C.
The Integrative Women's Health Institute
support@integrativewomenshealthinstitute.com
http://integrativewomenshealthinstitute.com

DEENA GOODMAN, P.T., W.C.S., B.C.B.-P.M.D.
Goodman Physical Therapy, Inc., West Los Angeles, CA
310-441-1102
www.goodmanphysicaltherapy.com

STEPHANIE PRENDERGAST, M.P.T.
The Pelvic Health & Rehabilitation Center, clinics in Berkeley,
San Francisco, Los Gatos, and Los Angeles, CA,
as well as in Lexington, MA
424-293-2305 (Los Angeles clinic for Stephanie Prendergast)
www.pelvicpainrehab.com

TRACY SHER, M.P.T., C.S.C.S.
Sher Pelvic Health & Healing in Orlando, FL
407-900-2876
www.sherpelvic.com

AMY STEIN, P.T., D.P.T., B.C.B.-P.M.D., I.F.
Beyond Basics Physical Therapy, New York, NY
212-354-2622
www.beyondbasicsphysicaltherapy.com

Education

BRODA O. BARNES RESEARCH FOUNDATION: The Broda
O. Barnes, M.D., Research Foundation, Inc. is a not-for-profit
organization dedicated to education, research, and training in the
field of thyroid and metabolic balance.
203-261-2101
www.brodabarnes.org

PRICE-POTTENGER NUTRITION FOUNDATION: The Price-
Pottenger Nutrition Foundation is a nonprofit, tax-exempt
educational organization dedicated to the promotion of enhanced
health through awareness of ecology, lifestyle, health food
production, and sound nutrition. At its core are the landmark
works of Drs. Weston A. Price and Francis M. Pottenger, Jr.,
pioneers in modern research.
800-366-3748
https://price-pottenger.org

Nutritional Training

AMERICAN COLLEGE OF HEALTHCARE SCIENCES: Founded
in New Zealand in 1978, ACHS launched in the United States in
1989 and became the first accredited, completely online college
offering holistic health education, with certificate, diploma, and
undergraduate and graduate degree programs.
800-487-8839
www.achs.edu

BAUMAN COLLEGE HOLISTIC NUTRITION AND CULINARY
ARTS: Bauman College educates future leaders, thinkers, and
creators in the holistic nutrition and culinary arts professions
to support people in achieving optimal health and create a
paradigm shift in the way our world thinks about food. Their goal
is to change the way people consume food from convenience to
conscious eating. They provide students with a comprehensive

understanding of nutrition, culinary arts, and business practices to prepare them for career success.

707-795-1284

www.baumancollege.org

CERTIFIED CLINICAL NUTRITIONIST TRAINING: A CCN is a board-certified clinical nutritionist. The primary service provided by a CCN is educational: to optimize the experience of health through enhanced nutrition. The Clinical Nutrition Certification Board (CNCB) is a 501(c)(3) nonprofit tax-exempt certification agency that provides professional training, examination, and certification for healthcare organizations, specialty credentialing programs, and state license/certification examinations. The Certified Clinical Nutritionist (CCN) examination establishes reputable standards of excellence.

972-250-2829

www.cncb.org

CERTIFIED NUTRITION SPECIALIST TRAINING: A certified nutrition specialist (CNS) is an advanced nutrition professional. CNSs engage in science-based advanced medical nutrition therapy, research, education, and more, in settings such as clinics, private practice, hospitals, and other institutions, industry, academia, and the community. The CNS certification is held by clinical nutritionists, physicians, and other advance-degreed healthcare professionals with a specialty in nutrition.

202-903-0267

www.nutritionspecialists.org

FUNCTIONAL DIAGNOSTIC NUTRITION TRAINING: Functional diagnostic nutrition (FDN) is a holistic discipline that employs functional laboratory assessments to identify malfunctions and underlying conditions at the root cause of the most common health complaints. FDN embraces metabolic individuality and provides a systematic approach that allows you to achieve consistent, repeatable, and successful clinical outcomes.

858-386-0075

http://functionaldiagnosticnutrition.com

INSTITUTE FOR FUNCTIONAL MEDICINE: The Institute for Functional Medicine is a leader in functional medicine education. The institute offers physicians and other healthcare professionals a systems-based approach to the prevention, diagnosis, and comprehensive management of complex chronic disease.

    800-228-0622

    www.functionalmedicine.org

INSTITUTE FOR INTEGRATIVE NUTRITION: The IIN was founded in 1992 by Joshua Rosenthal. Once a small classroom of passionate students in New York City, it is now the largest nutrition school in the world. Through its innovative online learning platform, the Institute for Integrative Nutrition has provided a global learning experience for more than 60,000 students and graduates in 122 countries worldwide.

    877-730-5444

    www.integrativenutrition.com

INSTITUTE FOR THE PSYCHOLOGY OF EATING: The Institute for the Psychology of Eating is a unique educational organization. Their mission is to forever change the way the world understands food, the body, and health. They offer trainings for professionals, programs for the public, online events, live workshops, and conferences as well as plenty of free online content and inspiration.

    info@psychologyofeating.com

    http://psychologyofeating.com

NUTRITIONAL THERAPY ASSOCIATION: As an education organization, the NTA is dedicated to helping individuals and healthcare professionals reverse the tragic and unsuspected effects of the modern diet based on the bioindividual nutritional needs of each patient. Throughout their training programs and seminars, students access a wide range of education tools and connect nationally with other practitioners in the healing arts. (Let them know Ann Louise sent you by using code ALG.)

    800-918-9798

    http://nutritionaltherapy.com

UNIVERSITY OF BRIDGEPORT: The University of Bridgeport's College of Naturopathic Medicine is committed to training physicians for the twenty-first century: doctors who are leaders in the emerging paradigm of health care, blending research and innovative technologies with the art of healing and natural therapeutics to provide patient-centered care.

800-392-3582

www.bridgeport.edu/academics/graduate/naturopathic
-medicine-nd

Professional Organizations

AMERICAN ACADEMY OF ANTI-AGING MEDICINE: The A4M is dedicated to the advancement of technology to detect, prevent, and treat aging-related disease and to promote research into methods to retard and optimize the human aging process. The A4M is also dedicated to educating physicians, scientists, and members of the public on biomedical sciences, breaking technologies, and anti-aging issues.

888-997-0112 or 561-997-0112

www.a4m.com

AMERICAN ACADEMY OF ENVIRONMENTAL MEDICINE: The American Academy of Environmental Medicine was founded in 1965 and is an international association of physicians and other professionals interested in the clinical aspects of humans and their environment.

316-684-5500

www.aaemonline.org

AMERICAN ASSOCIATION OF NATUROPATHIC PHYSICIANS (AANP): Naturopathic physicians are licensed in the following states: Alaska, Arizona, California, Colorado, Connecticut, District of Columbia, Hawaii, Kansas, Maine, Maryland, Minnesota, Montana, New Hampshire, North Dakota, Oregon, Utah, Vermont, Washington, United States Territories: Puerto Rico and Virgin Islands. For a referral to a naturopathic physician who can guide you with natural hormone therapy, you can contact:

202-237-8150

www.naturopathic.org

AMERICAN COLLEGE FOR ADVANCEMENT IN MEDICINE (ACAM): ACAM enables members of the public to connect with physicians who take an integrative approach to patient care and empowers individuals with information about integrative medicine treatment options. For a referral to a medical doctor or osteopath who is knowledgeable in the use of natural hormone replacement, you can contact:

800-532-3688

www.acam.org

INTERNATIONAL ASSOCIATION FOR COLON HYDROTHERAPY: I-ACT heightens the awareness of the colon hydrotherapy profession, ensures continuing and progressive education in the field of colon hydrotherapy, and offers a nationwide referral for people looking for a colon hydrotherapist.

210-366-2888

www.i-act.org

Testing and Labs

CELL SCIENCE SYSTEMS (PROVIDER FOR THE ALCAT TEST): The Alcat Test may help uncover which foods and other substances trigger chronic inflammation and its related health issues, such as gastrointestinal or metabolic disorders. The Alcat Test measures cellular reactions to more than 450 substances. Medical studies using the Alcat Test to guide diet have shown significant improvement of many common symptoms.

800-872-5228

https://cellsciencesystems.com

CYREX LABS: Cyrex Labs is an advanced clinical laboratory focusing on mucosal, cellular, and humoral immunology and specializing in offering antibody arrays for complex thyroid, gluten, and other food-associated autoimmunity testing.

877-772-9739

https://cyrexlabs.com

DIAGNOS-TECHS: Founded in 1987, Diagnos-Techs has been a pioneer and leader in offering salivary hormone testing and a complete GI panel for parasites, bacteria, and microbiome imbalances. Their commitment to assisting healthcare professionals in restoring patients' health and wellness is impressive, with more than 1.2 million specimens tested per year.

425-251-0596

www.diagnostechs.com

ELISA/ACT BIOTECHNOLOGIES: ELISA/ACT Biotechnologies is an exclusive provider of high-sensitivity lymphocyte response assay tests, the gold standard in delayed hypersensitivity testing.

800-553-5472

www.elisaact.com

IMMUNO LABORATORIES: Immuno Laboratories in Fort Lauderdale, Florida, is widely recognized as one of the leading food and environmental allergy testing facilities in the world. Since its inception, the company has conducted more than thirty-three million food sensitivity tests with 97 percent of its physicians testing for ten years or more—a clear indication of physician and patient satisfaction.

800-231-9197

www.immunolabs.com

MERIDIAN VALLEY LAB: Meridian Valley Lab is a leader in allergy and hormone testing, specializing in comprehensive twenty-four-hour urine hormone and metabolite testing. Meridian Valley was the first lab in the United States to offer this test to help doctors use bioidentical hormone replacement therapy safely and effectively.

206-209-4200

http://meridianvalleylab.com

TRACE ELEMENTS, INC.: Trace Elements is an independent testing laboratory specializing in hair tissue mineral analysis (HTMA) for healthcare professionals worldwide. With continued growth since its inception in 1984, Trace Elements serves thousands of health professionals of all specialties in more than forty-six countries.

  800-824-2314

  www.traceelements.com

ZRT LABORATORY: Founded by David Zava, ZRT is a CLIA certified diagnostic laboratory and the leader in hormone and wellness testing, providing accurate and meaningful test results that assist healthcare providers in making informed treatment decisions.

  866-600-1636

  www.zrtlab.com

Magazines and Newsletters

FIRST FOR WOMEN MAGAZINE: With an understanding that women have busy lives, *First for Women* delivers helpful tips and credible information you can't get anywhere else. The magazine provides numerous motivational articles on living a well-rounded life, nurturing family, owning a pet, preparing healthy menus, and just having fun! *First for Women* is very visual, with lots of quick tips and advice that make it easy to read as your schedule allows. I am proud to be a regular contributor.

  201-569-6699

  www.firstforwomen.com

HEALTH SCIENCES INSTITUTE (HSI) NEWSLETTER: HSI is an independent organization, dedicated to uncovering and researching the most urgent advances in modern underground medicine. As a member of the professional advisory panel, I can verify that this cutting-edge newsletter is devoted to presenting extraordinary products to its members before the products hit the marketplace. They were the first to break the Ultra H-3 story—the extraordinary product for arthritis, depression, and antiaging. The Health Sciences Institute provides private access to hidden cures, powerful discoveries, breakthrough treatments, and advances in modern underground medicine.

888-213-0764

http://hsionline.com

NUTRITION & HEALING NEWSLETTER: As an author of nine books on everything from thyroid disorders to back pain, Dr. Glenn S. Rothfeld has helped thousands of patients find lasting solutions to even the most stubborn health problems. These latest health discoveries are now available each month by subscribing to Dr. Rothfeld's *Nutrition & Healing* newsletter.

http://nutritionandhealing.com

NUTRITION NEWS: Siri Khalsa is a wonderful veteran journalist who has been in the business of providing health education for more than twenty-five years. Her engaging blog covers a wide variety of contemporary and current topics, and you can receive her monthly online newsletter by subscribing.

www.nutritionnews.com

TASTE FOR LIFE MAGAZINE: *Taste for Life* magazines can be found in health food stores, natural product chains, food co-ops, and supermarkets nationwide. Their publication offers excellent articles on pertinent health issues and provides readers an informative educational source on a variety of levels. I am proud to sit on *Taste for Life*'s editorial board. Their online website is also a one-stop natural health resource.

603-283-0034

www.tasteforlife.com

TOTAL HEALTH ONLINE MAGAZINE: The mission of *Total Health* online magazine is to advocate self-managed natural health, emphasize the importance of becoming the cocaptain of your own healthcare team, and address the imperatives to wellness. To achieve this, they provide you, the reader, with the information and resources needed to establish and maintain optimum health as well as to potentiate your immune system in times of crises. I am an associate editor for this outstanding publication.

http://totalhealthmagazine.com

TOTAL WELLNESS NEWSLETTER: Dr. Sherry A. Rogers is certified by the American Board of Environmental Medicine, is a fellow of the American College of Allergy, Asthma, and Immunology and a fellow of the American College of Nutrition, and has more than twenty-five years of board certification by the American Board of Family Practice. Her monthly newsletter, *Total Wellness,* is designed to save her readers money in office visits by keeping folks abreast of the latest cutting-edge research and findings.

800-846-6687

https://prestigepublishing.com/products/total-wellness -newsletter

WOMEN'S HEALTH LETTER: Dr. Janet Zand, O.M.D., L.Ac., is a board-certified acupuncturist, a doctor of traditional Chinese medicine, a nationally respected author and lecturer, a natural health practitioner, and an herbal and nutraceutical products formulator who has helped thousands of people achieve better health. Dr. Zand is the editor-in-chief of this informative monthly newsletter.

800-791-3459

www.womenshealthletter.com

Pure Food and Clean Water

MEAT

AMERICAN FARMERS NETWORK will help you find 100 percent grass-fed, USDA certified organic steaks, beef, chicken, and more.

www.americanfarmersnetwork.com

AMERICAN GRASSFED is an organization of certified grass-fed meat producers.
877-774-7277
www.americangrassfed.org

COMMUNITY INVOLVED IN SUSTAINING AGRICULTURE (CISA) is dedicated to sustaining agriculture and promoting the products of small farms.
413-665-7100
www.buylocalfood.org

THE CORNUCOPIA INSTITUTE maintains web-based tools rating all certified organic brands of eggs, dairy products, and other commodities, based on their ethical sourcing and authentic farming practices, separating CAFO "organic" production from authentic organic practices.
608-625-2000
www.cornucopia.org

THE EAT WELL GUIDE site includes state-by-state listings of meat that is raised without antibiotics.
www.eatwellguide.org

EAT WILD provides lists of certified organic farmers known to produce safe, wholesome raw dairy products as well as grass-fed beef and other organic produce.
253-759-2318
www.eatwild.com

FOODROUTES NETWORK's "Find Good Food" map can help you connect with local farmers to find the freshest, tastiest food possible. On their interactive map, you can find a listing for local farmers, CSAs, and markets near you.
814-571-8319
http://foodroutes.org

THE GRASSFED EXCHANGE has a listing of producers selling organic and grass-fed meats across the United States.
256-996-3142
www.grassfedexchange.com

LOCALHARVEST will help you find good food close to you.
831-515-5602
www.localharvest.org

NATIONAL FARMERS MARKET DIRECTORY will help you find a farmers' market near you.
http://nfmd.org

WESTON A. PRICE has local chapters in most states, and many of them are connected with buying clubs in which you can easily purchase organic foods, including grass-fed raw dairy products like milk and butter.
202-363-4394
www.westonaprice.org

FISH

Sardines from Bela and Crown Prince are often carried in finer health food stores. But if not, here is the contact information for these two fine brands:

BELA SARDINES
617-245-0490
www.belabrandseafood.com/home

CROWN PRINCE
800-447-2524
www.crownprince.com

The following websites carry wild salmon, a rich source of the omega-3 fatty acids. Some have tested their fish and have found that they are virtually mercury-free.

COPPER RIVER SEAFOODS
907-522-7806
www.copperriverseafood.com

EAST POINT SEAFOOD MARKET
206-257-1486
www.eastpointseafood.com

ECOFISH
603-834-6034
www.ecofish.com

FISHING VESSEL ST. JUDE
425-378-0680
www.tunatuna.com

VITAL CHOICE WILD SEAFOOD & ORGANICS
800-608-4825
www.vitalchoice.com

WILD SALMON SEAFOOD MARKET
888-222-3474
http://wildsalmonseafood.com

ORGANICS

You can learn about organic food and organic farming from the following nonprofit organizations.

COMMUNITY ALLIANCE WITH FAMILY FARMERS
530-756-8518
www.facebook.com/famfarms

THE LAND INSTITUTE
785-823-5376
https://landinstitute.org

ORGANIC FARMING RESEARCH FOUNDATION
831-426-6606
http://ofrf.org

ORGANIC TRADE ASSOCIATION
202-403-8630
www.ota.com

WATER

CLEAN WATER REVIVAL: CWR specializes in custom-designed water filtration equipment, air purifiers, and survival and personal protection equipment.
7897 SW Jack James Drive, Suite C, Stuart, FL 34997
800-444-3563
www.cwrenviro.com

ENVIRONMENTAL PROTECTION AGENCY SAFE DRINKING WATER HOTLINE
800-426-4791
www.epa.gov/ground-water-and-drinking-water /safe-drinking-water-hotline

NATIONAL TESTING LABORATORIES, LTD.
800-458-3330
www.ntllabs.com

SUBURBAN TESTING LABS
800-433-6595
www.suburbantestinglabs.com

Other Resources

3GVIBRATION.COM (A DIVISION OF VITALITY HEALTH & FITNESS): Whole-body vibrational training was created by Bob Thomas in 1984. An osteoporosis-preventing exercise, it uses 3G Vibration platforms that vibrate at a specific speed to take advantage of gravity and trigger muscles to use their natural reflexive response. 3G Vibration is the source for all of your whole-body vibration equipment and training needs.

For ALG fans, 3G Vibration is offering special discounts on top of their sale prices!

For seniors, choose the AVT 3.0 Whole Body Vibration Machine. (Take $100 off using the code ANNLOUISE3 at checkout.)

For exercisers, choose the AVT 5.0 Deluxe Whole Body Vibration Machine. (Take $250 off using the code ANNLOUISE5 at checkout.)

For professionals or heavy-duty exercisers, choose the AVT 6.0 Professional Whole Body Vibration Machine. (Take $350 off using the code ANNLOUISE6 at checkout.)

855-777-8423

www.3gvibration.com

ASEA: Over time, due to aging, stress, and environmental toxins, our bodies lose the ability to function at optimum levels. ASEA Redox Supplement, suspended in a pristine saline solution, is composed of the same life-sustaining molecules that exist in the human body. It works at the cellular level to enhance function and assist your body's natural efforts to maximize energy and vitality. As the world's only supplement containing redox signaling molecules, ASEA can help reset health on a cellular level and aid in repair of the body's natural processes.

888-438-5971

www.aseaglobal.com

DEFENDERSHIELD: DefenderShield products guard against portable device radiation and heat that can possibly harm the body. They provide solutions that use conductive, nonconductive, and highly advanced absorption shielding materials that interwork in unison to block, divert, and absorb potentially dangerous EMFs of extremely low frequency (ELF) radiation, radio frequency (RF), and heat radiation.

800-499-2418

www.defendershield.com

HUMANSCALE: Humanscale makes products that allow workstations to adapt to the user, not the other way around. Founded in 1983 by CEO Robert King with a focus on high-performance tools that support a healthy, more active way of working, Humanscale is now a global ergonomics leader with a reputation for designing intuitive products that improve the comfort and health of office workers.

800-400-0625
www.humanscale.com

INTERNATIONAL INSTITUTE FOR BUILDING-BIOLOGY & ECOLOGY: IBE is a nonprofit North American organization that combines Bau-Biologie, ecological principles, and technical expertise to support healthy living and a more sustainable environment, according to the precautionary principle.

866-960-0333
http://hbelc.org

LESSEMF: Less EMF, Inc., provides a wide range of products—including EF and RF meters, Gauss meters, electrosmog detectors, and shielding devices—for identifying and protecting against electromagnetic pollution.

518-608-6479
www.lessemf.com

POWER PLATE: Whole-body vibration was first used by the cosmonauts to combat muscle and bone loss caused by extended stays in zero gravity. Today, Power Plate (known as advanced acceleration training) has continued developing the technology to create products and training programs that deliver legendary performance for professional sports teams, medical facilities, health clubs, studios, and individuals around the globe.

877-877-5283
http://powerplate.com

Selected References

"About Truth in Olive Oil." Truth in Olive Oil website. http://www.truthinoliveoil
.com/about-truth-olive-oil.

"About Varidesk." Varidesk website. http://www.varidesk.com/about-varidesk.

Abrahamson, E. M., and A. W. Pezet. *Body, Mind and Sugar*. New York: Holt,
Rinehart, 1951.

"Adipose Tissue (from *Wikipedia*)." Science Daily. http://www.sciencedaily.com
/terms/adipose_tissue.htm.

Aesoph, Lauri. "Body Wise: Health Alert for Women." *Delicious!* October 1996, 26–30.

The Alternative Daily. "Grains vs. Seeds: What's the Scoop?" http://www.the
alternativedaily.com/grains-vs-seeds-whats-the-scoop.

Ameer, B., R. A. Weintraub, J. V. Johnson, R. A. Yost, and R. L. Rouseff. "Flavanone
Absorption After Naringin, Hesperidin, and Citrus Administration." *Clinical
Pharmacology and Therapeutics* 60, no. 1 (1996): 34–40.

American Chemistry Council. *The Benefits of Chlorine Chemistry in Water Treatment*.
December 2008. http://yosemite.epa.gov/sab%5CSABPRODUCT.nsf/EC591C83
E0AE1B5A852579670071541A/$File/ATT4WSEA.pdf.

American Institute for Cancer Research. "AICR's Foods That Can Fight Cancer:
Flaxseed." http://www.aicr.org/foods-that-fight-cancer/flaxseed.html#research.

American Psychological Association. "Report Highlights: *2015 Stress in America*."
http://www.apa.org/news/press/releases/stress/2015/highlights.aspx.

American Psychological Association. "Stress: The Different Kinds of Stress."
http://www.apa.org/helpcenter/stress-kinds.aspx.

American Society for Reproductive Medicine. *Menopause and Perimenopause*. Patient
Information Series, 1992.

"Amino Acids." Medline Plus. U.S. National Library of Medicine. Last modified
March 9, 2017. http://www.nlm.nih.gov/medlineplus/ency/article/002222.htm.

Anderson, Charlotte Hilton. "8 Benefits of High-Intensity Interval Training (HIIT)."
Shape. http://www.shape.com/fitness/workouts/8-benefits-high-intensity
-interval-training-hiit.

Andreassi, M., P. Forleo, A. Di Lorio, S. Masci, G. Abate, and P. Amerio. "Efficacy
of Gamma Linolenic Acid in the Treatment of Patients with Atopic Dermatitis."
Journal of International Medical Research 25, no. 5 (1997): 266–74.

Andrews, Edmund L. "In Victory for U.S., Europe Ban on Treated Beef Is Ruled
Illegal." *New York Times*, May 9, 1997. http://www.nytimes.com/1997/05/09
/business/in-victory-for-us-europe-ban-on-treated-beef-is-ruled-illegal.html.

Angier, Natalie. "New Respect for Estrogen's Influence." *New York Times*, June 24,
1997. http://www.nytimes.com/1997/06/24/science/new-respect-for-estrogen-s
-influence.html.

Anjali. "The Truth About Calories and Calorie Counting." *The Picky Eater* [blog]. October 21, 2015. http://pickyeaterblog.com/the-truth-about-calories-and -calorie-counting.

Anne, Melodie. "Food Sources of Glucose." Livestrong.com. Last modified February 18, 2014. http://www.livestrong.com/article/100663-sources-glucose.

Arisaka M., O. Arisaka, and Y. Yamashiro. "Fatty Acid and Prostaglandin Metabolism in Children with Diabetes Mellitus. II. The Effect of Evening Primrose Oil Supplementation on Serum Fatty Acid and Plasma Prostaglandin Levels." *Prostaglandins, Leukotrienes, and Essential Fatty Acids* 43, no. 3 (1991): 197–201.

Asp, Karen. "Superwoman Syndrome Fuels Pill-Pop Culture." NBCNews.com. Last modified February 24, 2010. http://www.nbcnews.com/id/35526012/ns/health -behavior/#.V5Dtn1fBTFI.

Associated Press. "Benefits Are Found in Asian Fish Diet." *New York Times,* August 1, 1997. http://www.nytimes.com/1997/08/01/us/benefits-are-found-in-asian-fish -diet.html.

Associated Press. "Female Jobseekers Face 'Superwoman Squeeze.'" *Bangor Daily News,* June 2, 1981. http://news.google.com/newspapers?nid=2457&dat =19810602&id=qgxbAAAAIBAJ&sjid=QE4NAAAAIBAJ&pg=1285,591231 &hl=en.

Baggerly, Carole. "The IOM Got It Wrong!" GrassrootsHealth.net. January 21, 2015. http://grassrootshealth.net/the-iom-got-it-wrong.

Bahmer, F. A., and J. Schäfer. "Treatment of Atopic Dermatitis with Borage Seed Oil (Glandol)—A Time Series Analysis Study [in German]." *Aktuelle Dermatologie* 18, no. 3 (1992): 85–88.

Bauer, P. M., P. C. M. Van de Kerkhof, and R. Maassen-de Grood. "Epidermal Hyperproliferation Following Induction of Microabscesses of Leukotriene B4." *British Journal of Dermatology* 114, no. 4 (1986): 409–12.

Berfield, Susan. "Inside Chipotle's Contamination Crisis." Bloomberg Businessweek. December 22, 2015. http://www.bloomberg.com/features/2015-chipotle-food -safety-crisis.

Bergland, Christopher. "Cortisol: Why 'The Stress Hormone' Is Public Enemy No. 1." *Psychology Today* online, January 22, 2013. http://www.psychologytoday .com/blog/the-athletes-way/201301/cortisol-why-the-stress-hormone-is-public -enemy-no-1.

Berkarda, B., H. Koyuncu, G. Soybir, and F. Baykut. "Inhibitory Effect of Hesperidin on Tumor Initiation and Promotion in Mouse Skin." *Research in Experimental Medicine* (Berlin) 198, no. 2 (1998): 93–99.

Berkeley Wellness. "Hydrogenated Oils." University of California. October 1, 2011. http://www.berkeleywellness.com/healthy-eating/food/article /hydrogenated-oils.

Bertomeu, M. C., G. L. Crozier, T. A. Haas, M. Fleith, and M. R. Buchanan. "Selective Effects of Dietary Fats on Vascular 12-HODE Synthesis and Platelet/Vessel Wall Interactions." *Thrombosis Research* 59, no. 3 (1990): 819–30.

Beutler, Jade. "High in Lignan Flax Oil." *Health Perspectives* 3, no. 2 (1997): 1–2.

BH Staff. "Tea and Fluoride . . . Beware of Fluoride." Beyond Health News. March 2, 2011. http://www.beyondhealthnews.com/wpnews/index.php/2011/03/tea -and-fluoride-beware-of-fluoride.

Blankenship, J., M. Crane, T. Mullen, R. Gregory, R. Lukens, and C. Sample. "Lipoprotein (a) Concentrations Increased on Vegan Type Diet with Powdered Soy Milk." *American Journal of Clinical Nutrition* 70, no. 3 (1999): 630s–32s. http://ajcn.nutrition.org/content/70/3/630s.full#sec-3.

Bloom, Marc. "Gain Without Pain: Fitness a Dose at a Time." *New York Times,* June 22, 1997. http://www.nytimes.com/1997/06/22/health/gain-without-pain -fitness-a-dose-at-a-time.html.

Bok, S. H., S. H. Lee, Y. B. Park, K. H. Bae, K. H. Son, T. S. Jeong, and M. S. Choi. "Plasma and Hepatic Cholesterol and Hepatic Activities of 3-Hydroxy-3-Methyl -Glutaryl-CoA Reductase and Acyl CoA: Cholesterol Transferase Are Lower in Rats Fed Citrus Peel Extract or a Mixture of Citrus Bioflavonoids." *Journal of Nutrition* 129, no. 6 (1999): 1182–85.

Borreli, Lizette. "Benefits of Oatmeal: Why You Should Add the Power Food to Your High-Fiber Diet." MedicalDaily.com. April 9, 2015. http://www.medicaldaily.com /benefits-oatmeal-why-you-should-add-power-food-your-high-fiber-diet-328788.

Briden, Lara. "The Curious Link Between Estrogen and Histamine Intolerance." *Lara Briden's Healthy Hormone Blog.* January 13, 2016. http://www.larabriden.com /the-curious-link-between-estrogen-and-histamine-intolerance.

Brody, Jane E. "Drug Researchers Working to Design Customized Estrogen." *New York Times,* March 4, 1997. http://www.nytimes.com/1997/03/04/science/drug -researchers-working-to-design-customized-estrogen.html.

Brody, Jane E. "Trans Fatty Acids Tied to Risk of Breast Cancer." *New York Times,* October 14, 1997. http://www.nytimes.com/1997/10/14/science/trans-fatty-acids -tied-to-risk-of-breast-cancer.html.

Brooks, J., W. E. Ward, J. Hilditch, J. Lewis, L. Nickell, and E. Wong. "Flaxseed, But Not Soy, Significantly Altered Urinary Estrogen Metabolite Excretion in Healthy Post-Menopausal Women." *FASEB Journal* 16, no. 5 (2002): A1005.

Brown, N. A., A. J. Bron, J. J. Harding, and H. M. Dewar. "Nutrition Supplements and the Eye." *Eye* (London) 12, pt. 1 (1998): 127–33.

Brown, Susan E. "How to Increase Spinal Bone Density with Exercise." *Better Bones* [blog]. May 13, 2016. http://www.betterbones.com/blog/post/how-to-increase -spinal-bone-density-with-exercise.

Brush, M. G., S. J. Watson, D. F. Horrobin, and M. S. Manku. "Abnormal Essential Fatty Acid Levels in Plasma of Women with Premenstrual Syndrome." *American Journal of Obstetrics and Gynecology* 150, no. 4 (1984): 363–66.

Bryant, Charles W. "What Are the Physical Effects of Stress?" HowStuffWorks.com. October 23, 2008. http://health.howstuffworks.com/wellness/stress-management /physical-effects-of-stress.htm.

Bulletproof. "The Bulletproof Guide to Omega 3 vs. Omega 6 Fats." http://www.bullet proofexec.com/omega-3-vs-omega-6-fat-supplements.

Burnard, S. L., E. J. McMurchie, W. R. Leifert, G. S. Patton, R. Muggli, D. Raederstorff, and R. J. Head. "Cilazapril and Dietary Gamma-Linolenic Acid Prevent the Deficit in Sciatic Nerve Conduction Velocity in the Streptozotocin Diabetic Rat." *Journal of Diabetic Complications* 12, no. 2 (1998): 65–73.

Caetano-Lopes, J., H. Canhão, and J. E. Fonseca. "Osteoblasts and Bone Formation." *Acta Reumatológica Portuguesa* 32, no. 2 (2007): 103–10. http://www.ncbi.nlm.nih .gov/pubmed/17572649.

Calderone, Julia. "The Rise of All-Purpose Antidepressants." *Scientific American* online, November 1, 2014. http://www.scientificamerican.com/article/the-rise -of-all-purpose-antidepressants.

Caldwell, L. "Is Male Menopause Myth or Reality?" *Men's Fitness,* July 1994, 102–4.

Carnahan, Jill. "Zonulin: A Discovery That Changed the Way We View Inflammation, Autoimmune Disease, and Cancer." JillCarnahan.com. July 14, 2013. http://www .jillcarnahan.com/2013/07/14/zonulin-leaky-gut.

Cassidy, A., S. Bingham, and K. D. R. Setchell. "Biological Effects of a Diet Rich in Isoflavones on the Menstrual Cycle of Premenopausal Women." *American Journal of Clinical Nutrition* 60, no. 3 (1994): 333–40.

Celiac Disease Foundation. "Sources of Gluten." http://celiac.org/live-gluten-free /glutenfreediet/sources-of-gluten.

Celiac Disease Foundation. "What Is Gluten?" http://celiac.org/live-gluten-free /glutenfreediet/what-is-gluten.

Center for Science in the Public Interest. "Q&A About Trans Fat and Hydrogenated Oils." May 18, 2004. http://cspinet.org/new/pdf/trans_q_a.pdf.

Centers for Disease Control and Prevention. "Drinking Water: Disinfection with Chlorine." U.S. Department of Health and Human Services. http://www.cdc.gov /healthywater/drinking/public/chlorine-disinfection.html.

Centers for Disease Control and Prevention. *National Diabetes Statistics Report: Estimates of Diabetes and Its Burden in the United States, 2014.* Atlanta, GA: U.S. Dept. of Health and Human Services, 2014. http://www.cdc.gov/diabetes/data /statistics/2014statisticsreport.html.

Centers for Disease Control and Prevention, National Center for Health Statistics. *National Health Interview Survey 2000.* U.S. Department of Health and Human Services. Ann Arbor, MI: Inter-University Consortium for Political and Social Research [distributor], 2002. http://www.icpsr.umich.edu/icpsrweb/NACDA /studies/3381.

Centre for Studies on Human Stress (CSHS). "Understand Your Stress: Acute vs. Chronic Stress." Institut Universitaire en Santé Mentale de Montréal. http://www.humanstress.ca/stress/understand-your-stress/acute-vs-chronic -stress.html.

Christiano, Donna. "Hot Flashes at 39?" *McCall's,* September 1995, 58.

Colborn, T., D. Dumanoski, and J. P. Myers. "Exposure Is Ubiquitous." *Our Stolen Future* website. http://www.ourstolenfuture.org/NewScience/ubiquitous /ubiquitous.htm.

Colditz, G. A., S. E. Hankinson, D. J. Hunter, W. C. Willett, J. E. Manson, M. J. Stampfer, C. Hennekens, et al. "The Use of Estrogens and Progestins and the Risk of Breast Cancer in Postmenopausal Women." *New England Journal of Medicine* 332, no. 24 (1995): 1589–93.

Corey, Michele. "Methylation: Why It Matters for Your Immunity, Inflammation, and More." MindBodyGreen website. April 9, 2015. http://www.mindbodygreen .com/0-18245/methylation-why-it-matters-for-your-immunity-inflammation -more.html.

Coward, L., N. C. Barnes, K. D. R. Setchell, and S. Barnes. "Genistein, Daidzein, and Their Beta-glycoside Conjugates: Antitumor Isoflavones in Soybean Food from

American and Asian Diets." *Journal of Agricultural and Food Chemistry* 41, no. 11 (1993): 1961–67.

Cranton, Elmer. *Resetting the Clock*. New York: Evans, 1996.

Crawford, Nicole. "Stop Doing Kegels: Real Pelvic Floor Advice for Women (and Men)." Breaking Muscle. http://breakingmuscle.com/womens-fitness/stop-doing -kegels-real-pelvic-floor-advice-for-women-and-men.

Crayhon, Robert. *Robert Crayhon's Nutrition Made Simple*. New York: Evans, 1994.

Czapp, Katherine. "Magnificent Magnesium." Weston A. Price Foundation website. September 23, 2010. http://www.westonaprice.org/health-topics/abcs-of-nutrition /magnificent-magnesium/#sthash.a2sdR0tq.dpuf.

Dabbs Jr., J. "Salivary Testosterone Measurements: Collecting, Storing, and Mailing Saliva Samples." *Physiology & Behavior* 49, no. 4 (1991): 815–17.

D'Adamo, Peter J. *Eat Right 4 Your Type*. New York: G. P. Putnam's Sons, 1996.

Daniel, Jill. "The Nutrients You May Be Missing." *Walking*, January/February 1997, 28–30.

Daniel, Kaayla. "The Legacy of Dr. Hazel Parcels." Weston A. Price Foundation website. September 16, 2008. http://www.westonaprice.org/health-topics/the -legacy-of-dr-hazel-parcels/#sthash.EBboHfqc.dpuf.

Davis, William. "The Gliadin Effect." Dr. William Davis website. January 14, 2012. http://www.wheatbellyblog.com/2012/01/the-gliadin-effect.

Deans, Emily. "Magnesium and the Brain: The Original Chill Pill." *Psychology Today* online, June 12, 2011. http://www.psychologytoday.com/blog /evolutionary-psychiatry/201106/magnesium-and-the-brain-the-original-chill-pill.

Dees, C., J. S. Foster, S. Ahamed, and J. Wimalasena. "Dietary Estrogens Stimulate Human Breast Cells to Enter the Cell Cycle." *Environmental Health Perspectives* 105, suppl. 3 (1997): 633–36.

Diamond, Seymour. *The Hormone Headache*. New York: Macmillan, 1995.

Diezel, W. E., E. Schulz, M. Skanks, and H. Heise. "Plant Oils: Topical Application and Anti-Inflammatory Effects (Croton Oil Test)." *Dermatologische Monatsschrift* 179 (1993): 173.

Drago, S., R. El Asmar, M. Di Pierro, M. Grazia Clemente, A. Tripathi, A. Sapone, M. Thakar, et al. "Gliadin, Zonulin, and Gut Permeability: Effects on Celiac and Non-Celiac Intestinal Mucosa and Intestinal Cell Lines." *Scandinavian Journal of Gastroenterology* 41, no. 4 (2006): 408–19.

"Drugs and Supplements: Vitamin B6 (Pyridoxine)." Mayo Clinic online. Last modified November 1, 2013. http://www.mayoclinic.org/drugs-supplements /vitamin-b6/background/hrb-20058788.

Duke, James A. *The Green Pharmacy*. Emmaus, PA: Rodale, 1997.

Eaton, S. B., and M. Konner. "Paleolithic Nutrition: A Consideration of Its Nature and Current Implications." *New England Journal of Medicine* 312, no. 5 (1985): 283–89.

Editors. "Bile." Encyclopædia Britannica. Last modified May 17, 2016. http://www .britannica.com/science/bile.

Editors. "Calcitonin." Encyclopædia Britannica. Last modified May 5, 2015. http:// www.britannica.com/science/calcitonin-hormone.

Editors. "Catecholamine." Encyclopædia Britannica. Last modified December 21, 2009. http://www.britannica.com/science/catecholamine.

Editors. "Gluten." Encyclopædia Britannica. Last modified April 6, 2016. http://www
.britannica.com/science/gluten.

Elias, P., quoted in "The Compounder's Corner: Exotic Claims" by R. L. Goldberg.
Drug and Cosmetic Industry 152, no. 1 (January 1993): 40.

Eliaz, Isaac. "Breast Health: Your Breast Health Questions, Answered." Better
Nutrition.com, October 2015. http://www.betternutrition.com/breast-health.

Emin, J. A., A. B. Oliveira, and A. J. Lapa. "Pharmacological Evaluation of the Anti-
Inflammatory Activity of a Citrus Bioflavonoid, Hesperidin, and the Isoflavonoids
Duartin and Claussequinone in Rats and Mice." *Journal of Pharmacy and
Pharmacology* 46, no. 2 (1994): 118–22.

Enig, Mary G. *Know Your Fats.* Silver Springs, MD: Bethesda Press, 2000, 85.

Environmental Working Group. "All 48 Fruits and Vegetables with Pesticide Residue
Data." 2017. http://www.ewg.org/foodnews/list.php.

Eskin, B. A., D. G. Bartuska, M. R. Dunn, G. Jacob, and M. B. Dratman. "Mammary
Gland Dysplasia in Iodine Deficiency." *Journal of the American Medical
Association* 200, no. 8 (1967): 115–19.

"Estriol and Triestrogen: Safe Methods of Estrogen Replacement Therapy." *Women's
Health Connections,* April/May 1994.

Euan, Monet. "Balancing Your Hormones Through Diet and Lifestyle." *Price-
Pottenger Journal* 39, no. 4 (2016): 14.

Fan, Y. Y., K. S. Ramos, and R. S. Chapkin. "Dietary Gamma-Linolenic Acid Enhances
Mouse Macrophage-Derived Prostaglandin E1 Which Inhibits Vascular Smooth
Muscle Cell Proliferation." *Journal of Nutrition* 127, no. 9 (1997): 1765–71.

Fasano, Alessio. "Zonulin and Its Regulation of Intestinal Barrier Function: The
Biological Door to Inflammation, Autoimmunity, and Cancer." *Physiological
Reviews* 91, no. 1 (2011): 151–75.

Feldman, Rachel. "Productivity Tips for Wearing the Superwoman Cape with Grace."
The Blog, *Huffington Post,* April 15, 2016. http://www.huffingtonpost.com/rachel
-feldman/wearing-the-superwoman-ca_b_9691774.html.

Finn, Kathleen. "Olive Oil Touted as Breast Cancer Preventive." *Delicious!* June 1995.

Finn, Kathleen. "26 Herbs for Better Health." *Delicious!* July 1996, 30–33, 65–67.

Fioretti, William C. "The Phytochemicals in Dioscorea Provide Support for the
Endocrine System." Proceedings of the 2nd Annual International Congress on
Alternative and Complementary Medicine, 1997.

FitDay Editor. "What Are Carbohydrates? An Easy to Understand Definition." FitDay
.com. http://www.fitday.com/fitness-articles/nutrition/carbs/what-are-carbo
hydrates-an-easy-to-understand-definition.html.

Fluoride Action Network. "Sources of Fluoride." FluorideAlert.org. 2017. http://
fluoridealert.org/issues/sources/tea.

Follingstad, Alvin H. "Estriol, the Forgotten Estrogen?" *Journal of the American
Medical Association* 239, no. 1 (1978): 29–30.

Fox, Maggie. "Olive Oil May Help Prevent Breast Cancer." NBCNews.com.
September 14, 2015. http://www.nbcnews.com/health/cancer/olive-oil-may
-help-prevent-breast-cancer-too-n426991.

FoxNews.com. "Blue Bell Creameries Issues Voluntary Recall of All Products After
Positive Listeria Test." April 21, 2015. http://www.foxnews.com/health/2015/04/21
/blue-bell-creameries-issues-voluntary-recall-all-products-after-positive.html.

Francis, Raymond. "Bouncing Magic." Beyond Health News. 2002. http://www
    .beyondhealthnews.com/articles/Rebounding.pdf.

Fuchs, N. K. "Calcium Controversy." *Natural Way,* April/May 1995, 12–14.

Fudyma, Janice. *What Do I Take? A Consumer's Guide to Non-Prescription Drugs.*
    New York: HarperPerennial, 1997.

Galati, E. M., M. T. Monforte, S. Kirjavainen, A. M. Forestieri, A. Trovato, and M. M.
    Tripodo. "Biological Effects of Hesperidin, a Citrus Flavonoid (Note I): Anti-
    Inflammatory and Analgesic Activity." *Farmaco* 40, no. 11 (1994): 709–12.

Galati, E. M., A. Trovato, S. Kirjavainen, A. M. Forestieri, A. Rossitto, and M. T.
    Monforte. "Biological Effects of Hesperidin, a Citrus Flavonoid. (Note III):
    Antihypertensive and Diuretic Activity in Rat." *Farmaco* 51, no. 3 (1996):
    219–21.

Garland, C. F., C. B. French, L. L. Baggerly, and R. P. Heaney. "Vitamin D
    Supplement Doses and Serum 25-Hydroxyvitamin D in the Range Associated
    with Cancer Prevention." *Anticancer Research* 31 (2011): 617–22. http://
    grassrootshealth.net/media/download/12928garland021811.pdf?utm_source
    =Newsletter+ONHA+Corrected+1%2F21%2F15&utm_campaign=Jan+21
    +2015+Newsletter&utm_medium=archive.

Garrison, Jayne. "Hormone Therapy: A New Option." *Health,* July/August
    1997, 106.

Genetic Science Learning Center. "Basic Genetics." Learn.Genetics. University of
    Utah. March 1, 2016. http://learn.genetics.utah.edu/content/chromosomes
    /telomeres.

Gittleman, Ann Louise. "A Vital Exercise Suited for Us All." AnnLouise.com. July 1,
    2016. http://annlouise.com/2016/07/01/a-vital-exercise-suited-for-us-all.

Gittleman, Ann Louise. *Beyond Pritikin.* New York: Bantam, 1988; rev. ed., 1996.

Gittleman, Ann Louise. *Eat Fat, Lose Weight.* Hayden Lake, ID: Blue Hills Publishing,
    2015. Kindle edition.

Gittleman, Ann Louise. "The Essential Six Female Nutrients." *Healthy Talk,* May
    1996, 1–8.

Gittleman, Ann Louise. *The Fat Flush Plan.* New York: McGraw-Hill, 2002.

Gittleman, Ann Louise. *The 40/30/30 Phenomenon.* New Canaan, CT: Keats, 1997.

Gittleman, Ann Louise. *How to Stay Young and Healthy in a Toxic World.* New York:
    McGraw-Hill, 1999.

Gittleman, Ann Louise. *Super Nutrition for Menopause.* New York: Pocket Books,
    1993.

Gittleman, Ann Louise. *Super Nutrition for Women.* New York: Bantam, 1991.

Gittleman, Ann Louise. *Your Body Knows Best.* New York: Pocket Books, 1996.

Gladwell, Malcolm. "The Estrogen Question." *New Yorker,* June 9, 1997, 54–61.

Goop. "The Secrets of the Pelvic Floor." http://goop.com/the-secrets-of-the-pelvic
    -floor.

Gottfried, Sara. *The Hormone Cure.* New York: Scribner, 2013.

Gottfried, Sara. *The Hormone Reset Diet.* New York: HarperOne, 2016.

Grady, Denise. "Diet-Diabetes Link Reported." *New York Times,* February 12, 1997.
    http://www.nytimes.com/1997/02/12/us/diet-diabetes-link-reported.html.

Graedon, Joe, and Teresa Graedon. *The People's Pharmacy.* Rev. ed. New York: St.
    Martin's Griffin, 1996.

Group, Edward. "What Is the *MTHFR* Genetic Defect and How Can It Affect You?" Global Healing Center. Last modified June 23, 2014. http://www.globalhealing center.com/natural-health/what-is-the-mthfr-genetic-defect.

Gunnars, Kris. "Why Modern Wheat Is Worse than Older Wheat." Authority Nutrition. http://authoritynutrition.com/modern-wheat-health-nightmare.

Haas, Robert. *Permanent Remissions.* New York: Simon & Schuster, 1997.

Hargrove, J. T., W. S. Maxson, and A. C. Wentz. "Absorption of Oral Progesterone Is Influenced by Vehicle and Particle Size." *American Journal of Obstetrics and Gynecology* 161, no. 4 (1989): 948–51.

Hawryluk, Markian. "The Unbeatable Brand: Premarin Topples the Odds Against Off-Patent Success." *Med Ad News* 14, no. 19 (1995).

Hayes, K. C., and A. Pronczuk. "Replacing Trans Fat: The Argument for Palm Oil with a Cautionary Note on Interesterification." *Journal of the American College of Nutrition* 29, suppl. 3 (2010): 253S–84S. http://www.ncbi.nlm.nih.gov/pubmed /20823487.

Herbert, Victor, and Genell Subak-Sharpe, eds. *Total Nutrition.* New York: St. Martin's Press, 1995.

Hill, E. E., E. Zack, C. Battaglini, A. Viru, and A. C. Hackney. "Exercise and Circulating Cortisol Levels: The Intensity Threshold Effect." *Journal of Endocrinological Investigation* 31, no. 7 (2008): 587–91.

Hoffman, Ronald. "Estrogen Dominance Syndrome." Ronald L. Hoffman, MD, website. October 4, 2013. http://drhoffman.com/article/estrogen-dominance -syndrome-2/#sthash.3gsitNIw.dpuf.

Holt, Stephen. "Phytoestrogens for a Healthier Menopause." *Alternative and Complementary Therapies* 3, no. 3 (2009): 187–93.

Hooper, Judith. "Does Menopause Really Begin in Your 30s?" *New Woman,* August 1997.

Horiuchi, T., K. Tanaka, and N. Shimizu. "Effect of Catecholamine on Aldosterone Release in Isolated Rat Glomerulosa Cell Suspensions." *Life Sciences* 40, no. 25 (1987): 2421–28.

"Hormone Tests: Blood Versus Saliva." *Women's Health Advocate* (newsletter) 3, no. 7 (1996): 1–2.

Horrobin, D. "Essential Fatty Acids in the Management of Impaired Nerve Function in Diabetes." *Diabetes* 46, suppl. 2 (1997): S90–3.

Horrobin, D. "The Role of Essential Fatty Acids and Prostaglandins in PMS." *Journal of Reproductive Medicine* 28, no. 7 (1983): 465–68.

Hutchins, Ken. *Super Slow: The Ultimate Exercise Protocol.* Ken Hutchins, 1992.

Hyman, Mark. *Eat Fat, Get Thin.* Boston: Little, Brown, 2016.

Iverson, L., K. Fogh, and K. Kragballe. "Effects of Dihomogammalinolenic Acid and Its 15-Lipoxgenase Metabolite on Eicosanoid Metabolism by Human Mononuclear Leukocytes In Vitro: Selective Inhibition of the 15-Lipoxygenase Pathway." *Archives of Dermatological Research* 284, no. 4 (1991): 222–26.

Jamal, G. A., and H. Carmichael. "The Effect of Gamma-Linolenic Acid on Human Diabetic Peripheral Neuropathy: A Double-Blind Placebo-Controlled Trial." *Diabetic Medicine* 7, no. 4 (May 1990): 319–23.

Jiang, W. G., R. P. Bryce, and R. E. Mansel. "Gamma Linolenic Acid Regulates Gap Junction Communication in Endothelial Cells and Their Interaction with Tumour

Cells." *Prostaglandins, Leukotrienes, and Essential Fatty Acids* 56, no. 4 (1997): 307–16.

Jiang, W. G., S. Hiscox, D. F. Horrobin, R. P. Bryce, and R. E. Mansel. "Gamma Linolenic Acid Regulates Expression of Maspin and the Motility of Cancer Cells." *Biochemical and Biophysical Research Communications* 237, no. 3 (1997): 639–44.

Johnson, M. M., D. D. Swan, M. E. Surette, J. Stegner, T. Chilton, A. N. Fonteh, and F. H. Chilton. "Dietary Supplementation with Gammalinolenic Acid Alters Fatty Acid Content and Eicosanoid Production in Healthy Humans." *Journal of Nutrition* 127, no. 8 (1997): 1435–44.

Ju, Y. H., C. D. Allred, K. F. Allred, K. L. Karko, D. R. Doerge, and W. G. Helferich. "Physiological Concentrations of Dietary Genistein Dose-Dependently Stimulate Growth of Estrogen-Dependent Human Breast Cancer (MCF-7) Tumors Implanted in Athymic Nude Mice." *Journal of Nutrition* 131, no. 1 (2001): 2853–59.

Keen, H., J. Payan, J. Allawi, J. Walker, G. A. Jamal, A. I. Weir, L. M. Henderson, et al. "Treatment of Diabetic Neuropathy with Gamma-Linolenic Acid. The Gamma-Linolenic Acid Multicenter Trial Group." *Diabetes Care* 16, no. 1 (1993): 8–15.

Key, T. J., G. B. Sharp, P. N. Appleby, V. Beral, M. T. Goodman, M. Soda, and K. Mabuchi. "Soya Foods and Breast Cancer Risk: A Prospective Study in Hiroshima and Nagasaki, Japan." *British Journal of Cancer* 81, no. 7 (1999): 1248–56.

King, Margie. *Nourishing Menopause*. New York: King Content Marketing, 2013.

King, Martha. "The Baby Boom Meets Menopause." *Good Housekeeping,* January 1992, 46–50.

Kockmann, V., D. Spielmann, H. Traitler, and M. Lagarde. "Inhibitory Effect of Steridonic Acid (18:4 n-3) on Platelet Aggregation and Arachidonate Oxygenation." *Lipids* 24, no. 12 (1989): 1004–7.

Koyuncu, H., B. Berkarda, F. Baykut, G. Soybir, C. Alatli, H. Gül, and M. Altun. "Preventive Effect of Hesperidin Against Inflammation in CD-1 Mouse Skin Caused by Tumor Promoter." *Anticancer Research* 19, no. 4B (1999): 3237–41.

Kresser, Chris. "The Little Known (But Crucial) Difference Between Folate and Folic Acid." Chris Kresser website. March 9, 2012. http://chriskresser.com/folate-vs -folic-acid.

Kresser, Chris. *Thyroid Disorders*. ebook. http://my.chriskresser.com/ebook/thyroid -disorders.

Kristof, Nicholas. "Are You a Toxic Waste Disposal Site?" *New York Times,* February 13, 2016. http://www.nytimes.com/2016/02/14/opinion/sunday/are-you-a -toxic-waste-disposal-site.html?_r=2.

Lam, Michael, and Dorine Lam. "Glandulars and Herbs for Adrenal Fatigue—Part 1." DrLam.com. http://www.drlam.com/blog/adrenal-fatigue-glandular-and-herbal -therapy-part-1/7544/#sthash.MUKu4IW3.dpuf.

Lark, Susan M. *The Estrogen Decision*. Los Altos, CA: Westchester, 1994.

Lark, Susan M. *Women's Wellness Today* (newsletter) 17, no. 4 (April 2010).

Laudan, Larry. *Danger Ahead*. New York: Wiley, 1997.

Laurence, Leslie. "What Women Must Know Before Menopause." *Ladies' Home Journal,* April 1994.

Laux, Marcus, and Christine Conrad. *Natural Woman, Natural Menopause*. New York: HarperCollins, 1997.

Lazarus, Richard S., and Susan Folkman. *Stress, Appraisal, and Coping*. New York: Springer, 1984.

Lee, John R. *Natural Progesterone: The Multiple Roles of a Remarkable Hormone*. Sebastopol, CA: BLL Publishing, 2000.

Lee, John R. *What Your Doctor May Not Tell You About Menopause*. New York: Warner Books, 1996.

Levy, Thomas E. *Death by Calcium*. Henderson, NV: Medfox Publishing, 2013.

Lipson, S. F., and P. T. Ellison. "Development of Protocols for the Application of Salivary Steroid Analysis to Field Conditions." *American Journal of Human Biology* 1, no. 3 (1989): 249–55.

Love, Susan M. *Dr. Susan Love's Hormone Book*. New York: Random House, 1997.

Love, Susan M. "Sometimes Mother Nature Knows Best." *New York Times*, March 20, 1997. http://www.nytimes.com/1997/03/20/opinion/sometimes-mother -nature-knows-best.html.

Majd, Sanaz. "Should You Drink Tap or Bottled Water?" QuickAndDirtyTips.com. June 4, 2015. http://www.quickanddirtytips.com/health-fitness/healthy-eating/know -your-nutrients/should-you-drink-tap-or-bottled-water#sthash.h07V5hjB.dpuf.

Manthorpe, R., S. Hagen Petersen, and J. U. Prause. "Primary Sjögren's Syndrome Treated with Efamol/Efavit. A Double-Blind Cross-Over Investigation." *Rheumatology International* 4, no. 4 (1984): 165–67.

Martin, W. "The Miracle of Evening Primrose Oil." *Townsend Letter for Doctors and Patients*, November 1992, 990–92.

Masley, Steven, and Jonny Bowden. *Smart Fat*. New York: HarperOne, 2016.

Matsuda, H., M. Yano, M. Kubo, M. Iinuma, M. Oyama, and M. Mizuno. "Pharmacological Study on Citrus Fruits. II. Anti-Allergic Effect of Fruit of Citrus Unshiu Markovich (2). On Flavonoid Components [in Japanese]." *Yakugaku Zasshi* 111, no. 3 (1991): 193–98.

Mayo Clinic. "Kegel Exercises: A How-To Guide for Women." September 25, 2015. http://www.mayoclinic.org/healthy-lifestyle/womens-health/in-depth/kegel -exercises/art-20045283.

McGowan, Mary P. *Heart Fitness for Life*. New York: Oxford, 1997.

"Medical Definition of Thyrocalcitonin." MedicineNet.com. Last modified May 13, 2016. http://www.medicinenet.com/script/main/art.asp?articlekey=16052.

"Medroxyprogesterone Acetate—Drug Summary." PDR. http://www.pdr.net/drug -summary/Provera-medroxyprogesterone-acetate-1015.

Meier, C., P. Trittibach, M. Guglielmetti, J.-J. Staub, and B. Müller. "Serum Thyroid Stimulating Hormone in Assessment of Severity of Tissue Hypothyroidism in Patients with Overt Primary Thyroid Failure: Cross Sectional Survey." *British Medical Journal* 326, no. 7384 (2003): 311–12.

"Melatonin." You and Your Hormones. Society for Endocrinology. Last modified January 16, 2015. http://www.yourhormones.info/Hormones/Melatonin.aspx.

Melnick, B., and G. Plewig. "Atopic Dermatitis and Disturbances in Essential Fatty Acid and Prostaglandin E Metabolism." *Journal of American Academy of Dermatology* 25, no. 5, pt. 1 (1991): 859–60.

Mercola, Dr. "Interesterified Fat—Is It Worse Than Trans Fat?" Mercola.com. March 5, 2009. http://articles.mercola.com/sites/articles/archive/2009/03/05/Interesterified -Fat--Is-it-Worse-Than-Trans-Fat.aspx.

Mercola, Dr. *Is Your Water Safe?: How Modern Water Sanitation Can Damage Your Health.* Mercola.com. http://mercola.fileburst.com/PDF/Chlorine-Special-Report.pdf.

Mercola, Dr. "Roundup and Glyphosate Toxicity Have Been Grossly Underestimated." Mercola.com. July 30, 2013. http://articles.mercola.com/sites/articles/archive/2013/07/30/glyphosate-toxicity.aspx.

Mercola, Dr. "Top Anti-Inflammatory Foods, Herbs, Spices." Mercola.com. February 2, 2015. http://articles.mercola.com/sites/articles/archive/2015/02/02/anti-inflammatory-foods-herbs-spices.aspx.

Messina, M., and S. Barnes. "The Role of Soy Products in Reducing Risk of Cancer." *Journal of the National Cancer Institute* 83, no. 8 (1991): 541–45.

Messina, M., and V. Messina. "Increasing Use of Soy Foods and Their Potential in Cancer Prevention." *Journal of the American Dietetic Association* 91, no. 7 (1991): 836–40.

Milligan, Patti Tveit. "Experience the Powerful Benefits of Soy." *Health Counselor,* August/September 1997, 57–59.

Miyake, Y., K. Yamamoto, N. Tsujihara, and T. Osawa. "Protective Effects of Lemon Bioflavonoids on Oxidative Stress in Diabetic Rats." *Lipids* 33, no. 7 (1998): 689–95.

"MoisturePom." PomHealth.com.

Mokdad, A. H., E. S. Ford, B. A. Bowman, D. E. Nelson, M. M. Engelgau, F. Vinicor, and J. S. Marks. "Diabetes Trends in the U.S.: 1990–1998." *Diabetes Care* 23, no. 9 (2000): 1278–83.

Montforte, M. T., A. Trovato, S. Kirjavainen, A. M. Forestieri, E. M. Galati, and R. B. Lo Curto. "Biological Effects of Hesperidin, a Citrus Flavonoid. (Note II): Hypolipidemic Activity on Experimental Hypercholesterolemia in Rat." *Farmaco* 50, no. 9 (1995): 595–99.

Morton, M. S., G. Wilcox, M. L. Wahlqvist, and K. Griffiths. "Determination of Lignans and Isoflavones in Human Female Plasma Following Dietary Supplementation." *Journal of Endocrinology* 142, no. 2 (1994): 251–59.

Murkies, A. L., C. Lombard, B. J. Strauss, G. Wilcox, H. G. Burger, and M. S. Morton. "Dietary Flour Supplementation Decreases Post-Menopausal Hot Flashes: Effect of Soy and Wheat." *Maturitas* 21, no. 3 (1995): 189–95.

Nachtigall, Lila E. "Too Young for Hot Flashes?" *Ladies' Home Journal,* July 1996, 110–14.

"New Study Supports Link Between Omega-3 Supplementation and Reduction in Depression." News release. Medical News Today. March 18, 2016. http://www.medicalnewstoday.com/releases/308070.php.

Nielsen, F. H., and J. G. Penland. "Boron Supplementation of Peri-Menopausal Women Affects Boron Metabolism and Indices Associated with Macromineral Metabolism, Hormonal Status, and Immune Function." *Journal of Trace Elements in Experimental Medicine* 12, no. 3 (1999): 251–61.

Nordqvist, Joseph. "Fish Oils Reduce Risk of Breast Cancer." Medical News Today. June 28, 2013. http://www.medicalnewstoday.com/articles/262612.php.

Northrup, Christiane. "Hormone Testing." *Health Wisdom for Women* (newsletter) 4, no. 7 (July 1997): 1–4.

Northrup, Christiane. *Women's Bodies, Women's Wisdom.* New York: Bantam, 1994.

O'Connor, Anahad. "Making a Case for Eating Fat." *Well* [blog]. *New York Times,* March 4, 2016. https://well.blogs.nytimes.com/2016/03/04/making-the-case -for-eating-fat/?_r=0.

Ornish, Dean. *Eat More, Weigh Less.* New York: HarperCollins, 1993.

Ovais, Mehreen. "The Superwoman Syndrome: A New Age Dilemma." *Express Tribune,* March 31, 2014. http://tribune.com.pk/story/688029/the-super-woman -syndrome-a-new-age-dilemma.

Palkhivala, Alison. "Glutathione: New Supplement on the Block." MedicineNet .com. June 30, 2001. http://www.medicinenet.com/script/main/art.asp?articlekey =50746.

Pelton, Ross, and Lee Overholser. *Revolution in Cancer Therapy.* New York: Fireside, 1994.

Perlmutter, David. "Learn: Science." David Perlmutter, MD, website. http://www .drperlmutter.com/learn/studies.

"Pica." Medline Plus. U.S. National Library of Medicine. Last modified March 9, 2017. http://www.nlm.nih.gov/medlineplus/ency/article/001538.htm.

Pitchrod, Paul. *Healing with Whole Food, Oriental Traditions, and Modern Nutrition.* Rev. ed. Berkeley, CA: North Atlantic Books, 1992, 77, 132–33, 288.

Pizzorno Jr., Joe. "Hydrogenated Oils and Trans Fats." *Integrative Medicine and Wellness* [blog]. WebMD. August 20, 2007. http://blogs.webmd.com/integrative -medicine-wellness/2007/08/hydrogenated-oils-and-trans-fats.html.

Posnick, Lauren M. "February/March 2002 Ask the Regulators—Bottled Water Regulation and the FDA." U.S. Food and Drug Administration. Last modified October 3, 2014. http://www.fda.gov/Food/FoodborneIllnessContaminants/Buy StoreServeSafeFood/ucm077079.htm (URL discontinued).

"Progesterone Cream or Pill—What's Best?" Virginia Hopkins Test Kits. http://www .virginiahopkinstestkits.com/progesterone_cream_or_pill.html.

"Prolamin." *Wikipedia.* Last modified September 19, 2016. http://en.wikipedia.org /wiki/Prolamin.

PsychTeacher(UK). "Stress Pathways." http://www.psychteacher.co.uk/stress/stress -pathways.html.

Pullman-Mooar, S., M. Laposata, D. Lem, R. T. Holman, L. J. Leventhal, D. DeMarco, and R. B. Zurier. "Alteration of the Cellular Fatty Acid Profile and the Production of Eicosanoids in Human Monocytes by Gamma-Linolenic Acid." *Arthritis and Rheumatism* 33, no. 10 (1990): 1526–33.

Raloff, Janet. "Hormone Therapy: Issues of the Heart." *Science News,* March 8, 1997, 140.

Ranabir, S., and K. Reetu. "Stress and Hormones." *Indian Journal of Endocrinology and Metabolism* 15, no. 1 (2011): 18–22. http://www.ncbi.nlm.nih.gov/pmc /articles/PMC3079864/#ref6.

Randall, Michael. "The Psychology of Stress: Cortisol and the Hypothalamic-Pituitary-Adrenal Axis." *Dartmouth Undergraduate Journal of Science* online. Fall 2010. http://dujs.dartmouth.edu/2011/02/the-physiology-of-stress-cortisol-and -the-hypothalamic-pituitary-adrenal-axis/#.V40zkVeJrVo.

"Rescue Remedy, Rescue Remedy Spray." BachFlower.com. http://www.bachflower .com/rescue-remedy-information.

Reuben, Suzanne H. *Reducing Environmental Cancer Risk: What We Can Do Now. Annual Report 2008–2009.* President's Cancer Panel (Laurel, MD: GPO, April 2010). http://deainfo.nci.nih.gov/advisory/pcp/annualReports/pcp08-09rpt /PCP_Report_08-09_508.pdf.

Robertson, Sally. "What Is DNA Methylation?" News-Medical.net. Last modified September 17, 2015. http://www.news-medical.net/life-sciences/What-is-DNA -Methylation.aspx.

Rose, D. P., M. Goldman, J. M. Connolly, and L. E. Strong. "High Fiber Diet Reduces Serum Estrogen Concentrations in Premenopausal Women." *American Journal of Clinical Nutrition* 54, no. 3 (1991): 520–25.

Rosenblatt, Robert A. "U.S. Agency Sounds Alarm About 'Miracle' Hormones." *Los Angeles Times,* April 28, 1997. http://articles.latimes.com/1997-04-28/news/mn -53319_1_hormone-supplements.

Rosenfeld, Isadore. "Health Report." *Vogue,* April 1997.

Ryan, George. *Reclaiming Male Sexuality.* New York: Evans, 1997.

Salmerón, J., J. E. Manson, M. J. Stampfer, G. A. Colditz, A. L. Wing, and W. C. Willett. "Dietary Fiber, Glycemic Load, and Risk of Non-Insulin-Dependent Diabetes Mellitus in Women." *Journal of the American Medical Association* 277, no. 6 (1997): 472–77.

Samsel, A., and S. Seneff. "Glyphosate, Pathways to Modern Diseases II: Celiac Sprue and Gluten Intolerance." *Interdisciplinary Toxicology* 6, no. 4 (2013): 159–84. http://www.ncbi.nlm.nih.gov/pmc/articles/PMC3945755.

Sapolsky, Robert. *Why Zebras Don't Get Ulcers.* New York: Holt, 2004.

Sathyamoorthy, N., T. T. Wang, and J. M. Phang. "Stimulation of PS2 Expression by Diet-Derived Compounds." *Cancer Research* 54, no. 4 (1994): 957–61.

Schofield, Lisa R. "A Balancing Act." *Whole Foods,* July 1997, 21–36.

Sears, Al. "PACE vs. HIIT." Al Sears, MD, website. http://www.alsearsmd.com/2014/10 /pace-vs-hiit.

Sears, Barry. *The Zone.* New York: ReganBooks, 1995.

Sellman, Sherrill. What Women Must Know. http://whatwomenmustknow.com.

Seppälä, Emma. "Benefits of Meditation: 10 Science-Based Reasons to Start Meditating Today." Emma Seppälä, Ph.D., website. http://www.emmaseppala .com/10-science-based-reasons-start-meditating-today-infographic/#.V5Jx _FfBRFI.

Serrin, Judith. " 'Superwoman' Complex a Pain in the Ego." *Boca Raton News,* July 28, 1976. http://news.google.com/newspapers?id=HsMPAAAAIBAJ&sjid=3IwDAAA AIBAJ&pg=7025,3342599&dq=superwoman-complex&hl=en.

Shandler, Nina. *Estrogen: The Natural Way.* New York: Villard, 1997.

Sheehan, Daniel M., and Daniel R. Doerge. Letter to Dockets Management Branch (HFA-305) of the Food and Drug Administration, February 18, 1999.

Shomon, Mary J. "Overview of Hypothyroidism." Sick to Death! website. http:// sick2death.com/facts-new.

Sinatra, Stephen S. *Optimum Health.* New York: Bantam, 1997.

"6 Things You Probably Didn't Know About Avocados." Healthy Living, *Huffington Post.* Last modified August 26, 2015. http://www.huffingtonpost.com/2015/08/26 /avocado-health-facts-didnt-dont-know_n_3786419.html.

Smith, C. J. "Non-Hormonal Control of Vaso-Motor Flushing in Menopausal Patients." *Chicago Medicine* 67 (1964): 193–95.

Society for Women's Health Research. "Hot Flash Havoc" Media Kit. April 2015. http://swhr.org/wp-content/uploads/2015/04/Hot-Flash-Havoc-Media-Kit_GENERAL.pdf.

"Soybeans Seem to Ease Menopause, Study Shows." *San Francisco Examiner*, November 11, 1996.

Spero, David. "What Is a Normal Blood Sugar Level?" Diabetes Self-Management. January 13, 2016. http://www.diabetesselfmanagement.com/blog/what-is-a-normal-blood-sugar-level.

Staff. "Tea: Fluoride." Linus Pauling Institute Micronutrient Information Center. Oregon State University. Last modified October 2015. http://lpi.oregonstate.edu/mic/food-beverages/tea#fluoride.

Stanford, J. L., N. S. Weiss, L. F. Voigt, J. R. Daling, L. A. Habel, and M. A. Rossing. "Combined Estrogen and Progestin Hormone Replacement Therapy in Relation to Risk of Breast Cancer in Middle-Aged Women." *Journal of the American Medical Association* 274, no. 2 (1995): 137–42.

Stolberg, Sheryl Gay. "Brand-New Recipe for Healthy Bones Adds More Calcium." *New York Times*, August 14, 1997. http://www.nytimes.com/1997/08/14/us/brand-new-recipe-for-healthy-bones-adds-more-calcium.html.

The Story of Stuff Project. "Story of Bottled Water FAQs." 2016. http://storyofstuff.org/story-of-bottled-water/story-of-bottled-water-faqs.

Sugar-Miller, Harriet. "Can Flaxseed Stave off Breast Cancer?" The Blog, *HuffPost Living Canada*. Last modified October 3, 2012. http://www.huffingtonpost.ca/harriet-sugarmiller/breast-cancer-flaxseed_b_1723226.html.

Sullivan, Karen, and C. Norman Shealy, eds. *The Complete Family Guide to Natural Home Remedies*. Rockport, MA: Element, 1997.

Szalay, Jessie. "Reference: What Are Carbohydrates?" LiveScience. August 25, 2015. http://www.livescience.com/51976-carbohydrates.html.

Talbott, Shawn M. "Chapter 7: Exercise." *The Cortisol Connection* website. From *The Cortisol Connection: Why Stress Makes You Fat and Ruins Your Health—And What You Can Do About It*. Alameda, CA: Hunter House, 2007. http://cortisolconnection.com/ch7_5.php (site discontinued).

Tanaka, T., H. Makita, K. Kawabata, H. Mori, M. Kabumoto, K. Satoh, A. Hara, et al. "Chemoprevention of Azoxymethane-Induced Rat Colon Carcinogenesis by the Naturally Occurring Flavonoids, Diosmin and Hesperidin." *Carcinogenesis* 18, no. 5 (1997): 957–65.

Tate, G., B. F. Mandell, M. Laposata, D. Ohliger, D. G. Baker, H. R. Schumacher, and R. B. Zurier. "Suppression of Acute and Chronic Inflammation by Dietary Gamma Linolenic Acid." *Journal of Rheumatology* 16, no. 6 (1989): 729–34.

Tate, G. A., and R. B. Zurier. "Suppression of Monosodium Urate Crystal-Induced Inflammation by Black Currant Seed Oil." *Agents and Actions* 43, nos. 1–2 (1994): 35–38.

Taylor. "What's Gluten?" *Gluten Away* [blog]. http://glutenaway.blogspot.com/p/allergy-symptoms.html.

Thompson, L. U., T. Li, J. M. Chen, and P. E. Goss. "Biological Effects of Dietary Flaxseed in Patients with Breast Cancer." 23rd Annual San Antonio Breast Cancer Symposium, December 6–9, 2000 (Abstract # 157).

Thompson, T. "Wheat Starch, Gliadin, and the Gluten-Free Diet." *Journal of the American Dietetic Association* 101, no. 12 (2001): 1456–59. http://www.ncbi.nlm .nih.gov/pubmed/11762742.

Tollesson, A., and A. Frithz. "Borage Oil: An Effective New Treatment for Infantile Seborrheic Dermatitis." *British Journal of Dermatology* 129, no. 1 (1993): 95.

University of Maryland Medical Center. "Black Cohosh." Last modified February 3, 2016. http://umm.edu/health/medical/altmed/herb/black-cohosh.

University of Maryland Medical Center. "Stress." Last modified January 30, 2013. http://umm.edu/health/medical/reports/articles/stress.

University of Wisconsin Hospital and Clinics Authority. "Health Facts for You: Fructose-Restricted Diet." April 2015. http://www.uwhealth.org/healthfacts /nutrition/376.pdf.

Upton, Arthur C., and Eden Graber, eds. *Staying Healthy in a Risky Environment: The New York University Medical Center Family Guide.* New York: Simon & Schuster, 1993.

USDA National Organic Program. *Introduction to Organic Practices.* U.S. Department of Agriculture. September 2015. http://www.ams.usda.gov/sites/default/files /media/Organic%20Practices%20Factsheet.pdf.

UVA Nutrition Services. *Low Fructose Diet.* University of Virginia Digestive Health Center. http://uvahealth.com/services/digestive-health/images-and-docs/low -fructose-diet.pdf.

Vaisey-Genser, Marion, and Diane H. Morris. *Flaxseed: Health, Nutrition, and Functionality.* Flax Council of Canada, 1997.

Valterra, Mikelann. "End the Superwoman Syndrome." DailyWorth. March 19, 2010. http://www.dailyworth.com/posts/382-end-the-superwoman-syndrome.

Vance, Sara. *The Perfect Metabolism Plan.* Newburyport, MA: Conari Press, 2015, 101.

Vanderhaeghe, Lorna R., and Karlene Karst. *Healthy Fats for Life.* Kingston, Ontario: Quarry Health Books, 2003, 4–5.

Vartak, S., R. McCaw, C. S. Davis, M. E. C. Robbins, and A. A. Spector. "Y-Linolenic Acid (GLA) Is Cytotoxic to 36B10 Malignant Rat Astrocytoma Cells but Not to 'Normal' Rat Astrocytes." *British Journal of Cancer* 77, no. 10 (1998): 1612–20.

Veugelers, P. J., and J. P. Ekwaru. "A Statistical Error in the Estimation of the Recommended Dietary Allowance for Vitamin D." *Nutrients* 6 (2014): 4472–75. http://grassrootshealth.net/media/download/veugelers_a_statistical_error -2014.pdf?utm_source=Newsletter+ONHA+Corrected+1%2F21%2F15&utm _campaign=Jan+21+2015+Newsletter&utm_medium=archive.

"Visceral Fat (Active Fat)." Diabetes.co.uk. http://www.diabetes.co.uk/body/visceral -fat.html.

Vliet, Elizabeth Lee. *Screaming to Be Heard.* New York: Evans, 1995.

Vozoff, Kate. "How to Handle the Menopause 'Unmentionable.'" *Townsend Letter for Doctors and Patients,* July 1996, 70–72.

Wallace, Edward C. "Homeopathy: Help for Hot Flashes." *Delicious!* October 1996, 32–35.

Walton, Alice G. "7 Ways Meditation Can Actually Change the Brain." Forbes.com. February 9, 2015. http://www.forbes.com/sites/alicegwalton/2015/02/09/7-ways -meditation-can-actually-change-the-brain/#77dd72607023.

Warga, Claire Landsberg. "Estrogen and the Brain." *New York,* August 11, 1997, 26–31.

Watts, David L. "Pre- and Post-Menstrual Syndrome." *Trace Elements, Inc., Newsletter* 3, no. 4, September/October 1989, http://www.traceelements.com/Docs/News%20 Sept-Oct%2089.pdf.

Watts, David L. *Trace Elements and Other Essential Nutrients.* Dallas: Trace Elements, 1995.

Wentz, Isabella. *Hashimoto's Thyroiditis.* Wentz LLC, 2013.

"What Is Theobromine?" Phytochemicals.info. http://www.phytochemicals.info /phytochemicals/theobromine.php.

Winslow, Ron. "Scientists See Promise in New Estrogen Drug." *Wall Street Journal,* August 20, 1997.

"Women's Health: A Special Section." *New York Times,* June 22, 1997.

Wright, Jonathan V. *New Secrets Every Woman Needs to Know.* Nutrition and Healing Library of Food and Vitamin Cures. Baltimore, MD: Healthier News, 2007. http://nutritionandhealing.com/wp-content/uploads/2009/05/woman.pdf.

Wright, Jonathan V., and John Morgenthaler. *Natural Hormone Replacement.* Petaluma, CA: Smart Publications, 1997.

Writing Group for the PEPI Trial. "Effects of Estrogen or Estrogen/Progestin Regimens on Heart Disease Risk Factors in Postmenopausal Women." *Journal of the American Medical Association* 273, no. 3 (1995): 199–208.

Yang, Z., S. Liu, X. Chen, H. Chen, M. Huang, and J. Zheng. "Induction of Apoptotic Cell Death and In Vivo Growth Inhibition of Human Cancer Cells by a Saturated Branched-Chain Fatty Acid, 13-Methyltetradecanoic Acid." *Cancer Research* 60, no. 3 (2000): 505–9.

Ziboh, V. A. "Lipoxygenation of Gamma Linolenic Acid by Skin Epidermis: Modulation of Epidermal Inflammatory/Hyperproliferative Processes." Proceedings of the Annual Meeting of the American Oil Chemists' Society, 1998, 25.

Ziboh, V. A., and M. P. Fletcher. "Dose-Response Effects of Dietary Gamma Linolenic Acid Enriched Oils on Human Polymorphonuclear-Neutrophil Biosynthesis of Leukrotriene B4." *American Journal of Clinical Nutrition* 55, no. 1 (1992): 39–45.

Ziboh, V. A., and C. C. Miller. "Essential Fatty Acids and Polyunsaturated Fatty Acids Significance in Cutaneous Biology." *Annual Review of Nutrition* 10 (1990): 433–50.

Zimmermann, M. B., and J. Köhrle. "The Impact of Iron and Selenium Deficiencies on Iodine and Thyroid Metabolism: Biochemistry and Relevance to Public Health." *Thyroid* 12, no. 10 (2002): 867–78.

"Zinc." The World's Healthiest Foods. http://www.whfoods.com/genpage.php?tname =nutrient&dbid=115.

Zurier, R. B., P. DeLuca, and D. Rothman. "Gammalinolenic Acid, Inflammation, Immune Responses, and Rheumatoid Arthritis." In *Gamma-Linolenic Acid: Metabolism and Its Roles in Nutrition and Medicine.* Edited by Y.-S. Huang and D. E. Mills. Champaign, IL: AOCS Press, 1996, 129–36.

Index

About the Author

Undisputedly the First Lady of Nutrition, Ann Louise Gittleman, Ph.D., C.N.S., is a *New York Times* bestselling author of more than thirty books on diet, detox, the environment, and women's health. Beloved by many, she is regarded as a nutritional visionary and health pioneer who has fearlessly stood on the front lines of holistic and integrative medicine. A Columbia University graduate, Gittleman has been recognized as one of the top ten nutritionists in the country by *Self* magazine and has received the American Medical Writers Association award for excellence and the Cancer Control Society Humanitarian Award. Visit her at AnnLouise.com.

Also by Ann Louise Gittleman

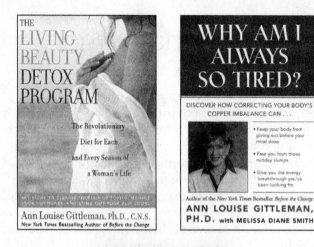

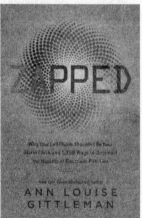